Current Practices in Ophthalmology

Series Editor
Parul Ichhpujani, Department of Ophthalmology, Government Medical College and Hospital, Chandigarh, India

This series of highly organized and uniform handbooks aims to cover the latest clinically relevant developments in ophthalmology. In the wake of rapidly evolving innovations in the field of basic research, pharmacology, surgical techniques and imaging devices for the management of ophthalmic disorders, it is extremely important to invest in books that help you stay updated. These handbooks are designed to bridge the gap between journals and standard texts providing reviews on advances that are now part of mainstream clinical practice. Meant for residents, fellows-in-training, generalist ophthalmologists and specialists alike, each volume under this series covers current perspectives on relevant topics and meets the CME requirements as a go-to reference guide. Supervised and reviewed by a subject expert, chapters in each volume provide leading-edge information most relevant and useful for clinical ophthalmologists. This series is also useful for residents and fellows training in various subspecialties of ophthalmology, who can read these books while at work or during emergency duties. Additionally, these handbooks can aid in preparing for clinical case discussions at various forums and examinations.

Adit Gupta • Prerana Tahiliani
Editors

Oculoplastic and Orbit Casebook

Springer

Editors
Adit Gupta
Mumbai Eye Plastic Surgery
Mumbai, Maharashtra, India

Prerana Tahiliani
Mumbai Eye Plastic Surgery
Mumbai, Maharashtra, India

ISSN 2523-3807 ISSN 2523-3815 (electronic)
Current Practices in Ophthalmology
ISBN 978-981-97-0595-5 ISBN 978-981-97-0593-1 (eBook)
https://doi.org/10.1007/978-981-97-0593-1

This Springer imprint is published by the registered company Springer Nature Singapore Pte Ltd.
The registered company address is: 152 Beach Road, #21-01/04 Gateway East, Singapore 189721, Singapore

Contents

About the Editors

Adit Gupta is consultant oculoplastic and orbit surgeon at Mumbai Eye Plastic Surgery, a dedicated ophthalmic plastic surgery center in Mumbai, India. He is an expert in the field of eyelid and facial cosmetic surgery. Over the past 8 years, he has performed several procedures for the cosmetic, structural, and functional rehabilitation of the eyelids and lacrimal region in India and the USA. Dr. Gupta completed his MD in ophthalmology from Advanced Eye Centre, PGIMER, Chandigarh, India following which he completed his oculoplastic fellowship at LV Prasad Eye Institute, Hyderabad, India. He pursued further training for his second fellowship in orbitofacial cosmetic surgery at the UCLA Stein Eye Institute, Los Angeles, California, USA under the tutelage of Dr. Robert Goldberg. In addition to eyelid surgery, Dr. Gupta focuses on cosmetic eyelid surgeries, thyroid eye disease, and revision procedures. Apart from clinical work, Dr. Gupta has keen interest in research, teaching, and developing minimally invasive techniques for orbital and cosmetic surgeries.

Prerana Tahiliani is consultant oculoplastic and orbit surgeon at Mumbai Eye Plastic Surgery and Lotus Eye Hospital, Mumbai, India. She completed her post-graduation in ophthalmology from Sri Sankaradeva Nethralaya, Guwahati, India followed by a fellowship in ophthalmic plastic surgery and ocular oncology at the LV Prasad Eye Institute, Hyderabad, India. During her tenure at LV Prasad, she developed a keen interest for ocular oncology and dacryology. She followed this up with a short stint at UCLA and CHLA, Los Angeles, USA in the year 2016. Dr. Tahiliani is a keen researcher and invited speaker at many national and international forums. Apart from this, she also is an avid teacher and likes encouraging the young leaders in oculoplastics.

Eyelid Lacerations and Canalicular Laceration

1

Varshitha Hemanth Vasanthapuram

1.1 Introduction

Eyelid lacerations form a major bulk of the ocular emergencies encountered in the Oculoplasty clinic. Periocular soft tissue trauma can range from a simple abrasion to avulsion, may be associated with orbital fractures/open globe injury or facial injury.

Eyelids play an important functional and aesthetic role. A good eyelid tear repair is crucial to preserve this. A thorough clinical examination and evaluation is paramount to effective surgical planning and repair.

1.2 Pre-requisites for a Good Surgical Planning

1.2.1 History

- Time since injury: Early repair is advocated, especially in laceration involving canaliculus.
- Mode of injury: It is important to note the mode of injury. For instance, in case of Road Traffic Accident (RTA) one must look for grease, gravel, stones, glass pieces within the laceration. In animal bite injury, anti-rabies vaccine and immunoglobulin need to be arranged. Other modes include assault, penetrating trauma related to occupation, blouse hook injury in babies, etc.

V. H. Vasanthapuram (✉)
Ophthalmic Plastic Surgery Services, Narayana Nethralaya, Bangalore, India

A. Gupta, P. Tahiliani (eds.), *Oculoplastic and Orbit Casebook*, Current Practices in Ophthalmology, https://doi.org/10.1007/978-981-97-0593-1_1

1.2.2 Clinical Assessment

The laceration should be assessed for the following:

- Full thickness or partial thickness.
- Eyelid avulsion.
- Extra-marginal/marginal involvement.
- Canthal involvement.
- Canalicular and lacrimal apparatus involvement.
- Soft tissue loss.
- Presence of foreign body.
- Additional injury—orbital fracture, globe injury.

1.2.3 Before the Surgery

- Pre- and post-operative photographic documentation.
- Proper patient communication and consent.
- Repair should be preceded by thorough saline and betadine wash.
- Tetanus toxoid injection and antibiotic coverage should be given.

Though the extent of periocular injury and cause is varied, following a general protocol can help in most occasions in the emergency room. This protocol should however be followed after a thorough assessment of the vitals, systemic status, and associated injuries.

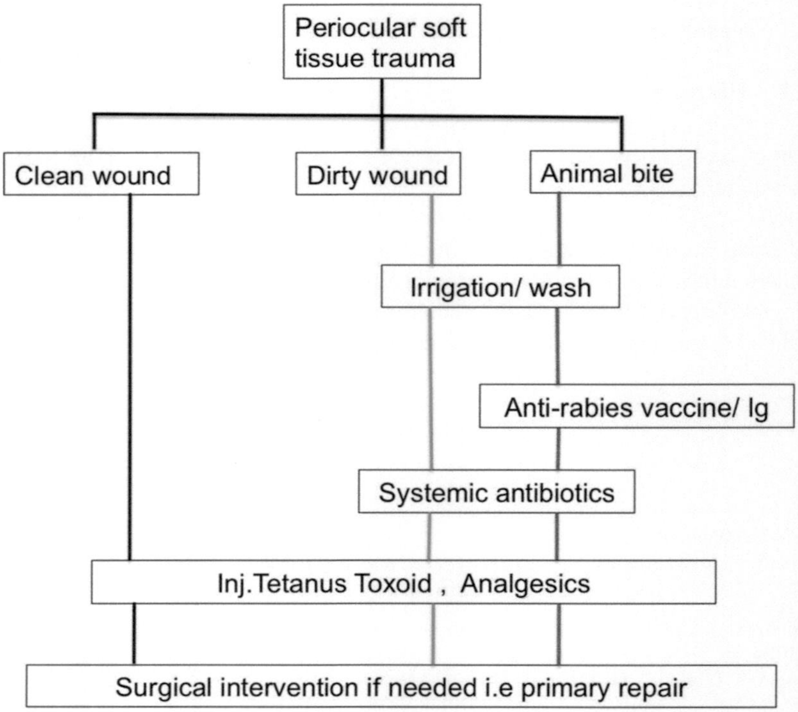

1.2.3.1 Irrigation

Soft tissue wounds less than 8 h old and surgical incisions are categorized as "clean" and wounds older than 8 h are categorized as "dirty" wounds [1]. Soft tissue injuries secondary to RTA may have mud, grease, gravel, glass pieces, etc. within the wound and vicinity. Cleaning and irrigation remove the dirt which aids in better assessment of wounds. Also, thorough irrigation reduces the organism load and decreases the risk of infection, especially in animal bites.

Irrigation of periocular soft tissue wounds at the author's institute is performed with normal saline solution, directly with the bottle in small wounds or with an intravenous (iv) infusion cannula attached to the bottle for large wounds. The nozzle is placed at a distance of approximately 1–2 inches from the wound. In case of grease or soil, gentle digital cleaning can aid. Wounds with associated globe injuries should be irrigated with caution.

Hollander et al. found that irrigation may not be beneficial in clean wounds. In fact, they cited irrigation deems the wounds more exposed to possible exogenous infection and trends towards worse cosmetic outcome after primary repair [2]. This was attributed to tissue trauma secondary to high pressure irrigation [2].

The author recommends gentle cleansing of clean wounds and irrigation of dirty wounds.

Wound debridement can be performed under anesthesia just before wound repair with an aim of maximum tissue preservation. The non-viable tissue can be excised and foreign bodies removed [3].

The periocular region has a rich blood supply. There can be bleeding from the supra-trochlear and supra-orbital vessels in lacerations involving the brow. Initial hemostasis can be achieved by pressure application.

1.2.3.2 Medications

Routine analgesics like non-steroidal anti-inflammatory drugs can be prescribed for pain. Topical broad-spectrum antibiotics should suffice for clean wounds [4]. In cases of animal bites, RTA, systemic immunosuppressed states such as diabetes, broad spectrum systemic antibiotics are recommended for 5–7 days [1, 4]. The author prescribes amoxicillin-clavulanate combination 30 mg/kg body weight iv or 625 mg orally (adults) at a twice daily dosing for 5 days.

Tetanus Immunization

Major wounds such as crush wounds, devitalized wounds, burns, fractures, avulsion, dirty wounds, and minor wounds such as scratches are prone to tetanus. It is vital to probe the history of prior tetanus immunization [5]. Tetanus administration for wounds as per the Advisory Committee on Immunization Practices (ACIP) recommendations is mentioned in Table 1.1 [6]. Tetanus toxoid (Tt) produces delayed immunity. Administering Tt in acute wounds does not provide the required immunity but ensures protection for future wounds, hence in cases of unknown immunization history or history of last booster in more than 10 years or greater than 5 years in case of contaminated wound, tetanus immune globulin (TIG) should be administered [5, 6]. The recommended TIG dosage for adult prophylaxis is 250–500 U IM in opposite extremity to Tt and 250 U IM in pediatric age group [5].

Table 1.1 Tetanus administration for wounds as per the Advisory Committee on Immunization Practices (ACIP) recommendations

History of adsorbed tetanus toxoid-containing vaccines (doses)	Clean, minor wound, DTaP, Tdap or Td[a]	Clean, minor wound, TIG[b]	All other wounds[c], DTaP, Tdap or Td[a]	All other wounds[c], TIG[b]
Unknown or <3	Yes	No	Yes	Yes
≥3	No[d]	No	No[e]	No

DTaP diphtheria and tetanus toxoids and acellular pertussis vaccine, *Tdap* tetanus toxoid, reduced diphtheria toxoid, and acellular pertussis, *Td* tetanus and diphtheria toxoids, *TIG* tetanus immune globulin

[a]DTaP is recommended for children <7 years of age. Tdap is preferred to Td for persons aged 11 years or older who have not previously received Tdap. Persons aged 7 years or older who are not fully immunized against pertussis, tetanus, or diphtheria should receive one dose of Tdap (preferably the first) for wound management and as part of the catch-up series; if additional tetanus toxoid-containing doses are required, either Td or Tdap vaccine can be used

[b]People with HIV infection or severe immunodeficiency who have contaminated wounds (including minor wounds) should also receive TIG, regardless of their history of tetanus immunizations

[c]Such as, but not limited to, wounds contaminated with dirt, feces, soil, and saliva; puncture wounds; avulsions; and wounds resulting from missiles, crushing, burns, and frostbite

[d]Yes, if ≥10 years since the last tetanus toxoid-containing vaccine dose

[e]Yes, if ≥5 years since the last tetanus toxoid-containing vaccine dose

1.2.4 General Principles in Repair

- Best performed under surgical loupe or microscope.
- Local infiltration or general anesthesia.
- Layered closure of tissues should be performed from deep to superficial.
- Skin suturing—eversion of wound edges during closure gives a better cosmetic outcome [4].
- Scarring along relaxed skin tension lines yields better results, hence the ragged edges of lacerations should be attempted to be converted to parallel edges to RSTL [4].
- Preserve as much soft tissue as possible during debridement [7].
- Avoid major reconstructive procedures during primary repair [7].
- Perform eyelid tear repairs after globe repairs in case of combined injuries.

Below are a few case scenarios illustrating the management of different grades of eyelid laceration.

1.3 Case Scenarios

1.3.1 Case 1

1.3.1.1 Case Summary

A 32-year-old female presented with trauma to the left eye following a fall from bicycle in the morning of her visit to the Eye Clinic. On examination, a full thickness laceration of the middle third of the left upper eyelid was noted (Fig. 1.1a). It was involving the margin, sparing the lateral canthus. The globe was intact. Visual acuity was 6/6 in both eyes, slit lamp examination was unremarkable.

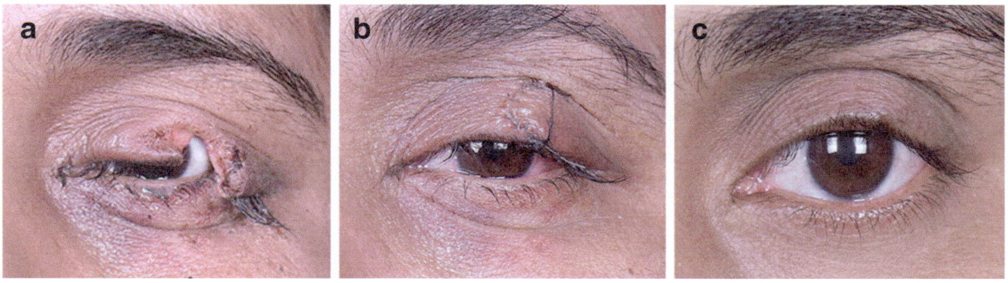

Fig. 1.1 (**a**) Full thickness upper eyelid laceration involving the margin; (**b**) immediate post-operative photograph; (**c**) appearance at post-operative 6 weeks

1.3.1.2 Case Management

This is a case of a margin involving full thickness laceration of the upper eyelid with no tissue loss. A good approximation and closure at the margin followed by layer-by-layer closure is required.

- The surgery was performed under local anesthesia.
- The lid margins were approximated and sutured with 6-0 silk (reverse cutting) vertical mattress suture. A good lid margin approximation is essential to a neat eyelid repair and avoid notching at the margin. An easy way to remember to take the bites is to follow the "near-near, far-far" rule (Fig. 1.2).
- The silk suture is passed along the line of the Meibomian gland (MG) openings. Needle is first passed at the level of second opening from the edge of the defect, through the tarsal plate of one edge of the defect then through tarsal plate at the other edge, bringing it out through the second MG opening from the other edge of the defect.
- Similarly, the next bite is passed through fourth Meibomian gland opening. The knot is tied at one end which is neither too tight nor too loose. The ends should be slightly pouting after knot. This ensures there is no notching after healing.
- After approximation of margin, layer-by-layer closure of tarsal plate is performed with 6-0 vicryl interrupted sutures with partial thickness bites.
- Next, the lash line is approximated and sutured with 6-0 vicryl simple interrupted suture.
- Orbicularis and skin are sutured with 6-0 vicryl (spatulated) interrupted suture (Fig. 1.1b).

1.3.1.3 Surgical Pearl

In cases of upper eyelid laceration extending beyond the tarsal plate, the LPS should be isolated and repaired to avoid blepharoptosis later.

1.3.1.4 Conclusion

Eyelid tears with margin defects should be well aligned with vertical mattress suture. The edge should be pouting slightly after tying the knot. Ensure the knot is of adequate tensile strength—neither tight nor loose. This avoids an eyelid notch (Fig. 1.1c).

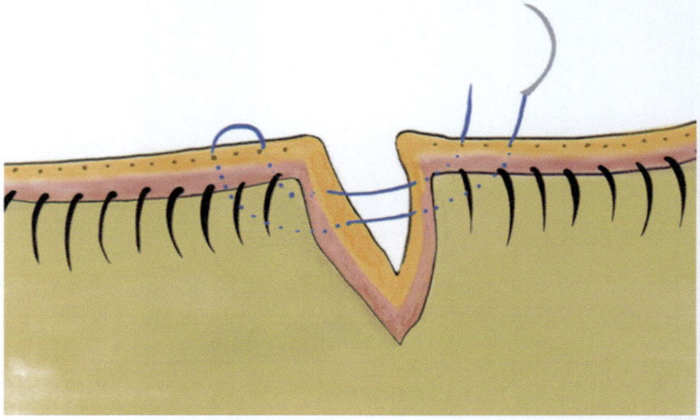

Fig. 1.2 Line diagram showing the passage of vertical mattress suture through the tarsal plate in marginal tear repair

1.3.2 Case 2

1.3.2.1 Case Summary

A 40-year-old gentleman presented with complaint of dog bite injury to his left eye 1 day back. On examination, there were three lacerations on the left upper eyelid—a full thickness laceration involving the upper canaliculus medially, a central partial thickness marginal tear and a full thickness marginal tear laterally (Fig. 1.3a and b). The globe was intact, rest of the eye examination was within normal limits. There was no additional facial injury.

1.3.2.2 Case Management

- This is a case of animal bite injury, as per WHO guidelines, this injury falls under Category III and hence post-exposure prophylaxis (PEP) should be provided. The PEP schedule is given in Table 1.2.
- In addition to vaccination, Rabies Immunoglobulin (RIG) should also be given at the dose of 20 IU/kg to provide passive immunity.
- The case was taken up under local anesthesia. A thorough saline and betadine irrigation was performed.
- Upper canalicular repair was performed first with mini-Monoka intubation under microscope (detailed description in Chap. 2).
  - Under microscope/surgical loupe, identify the proximal and distal ends of the injured canaliculus—look for the Calamari sign. (Can use intra-op Alphagan eye drops to enhance visibility or inject dye through the opposite canaliculus).
  - Check for the appropriate length of the mini-Monoka stent and cut.
  - Insert the stent through the punctum using blunt forceps and through the lacerated ends of the canaliculus.
  - Place marginal sutures.
  - Repair and approximate the rest of the tissues layer by layer with 6-0 vicryl (spatulated) interrupted sutures.

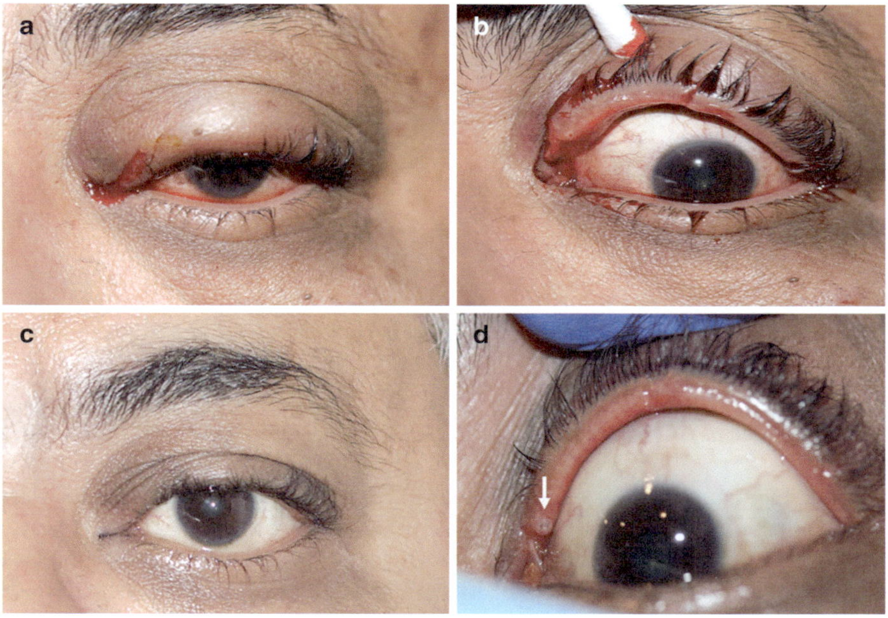

Fig. 1.3 (**a**) Left upper eyelid laceration involving the upper canaliculus; (**b**) upper eyelid retracted showing the lacerated upper canaliculus, marginal tear at middle third and laterally; (**c**) appearance at post-operative 6 weeks showing healed upper eyelid with good contour; (**d**) the mini-Monoka stent in place (arrow)

- Next the lateral marginal tear was repaired with 6-0 silk reverse cutting, vertical mattress suture (detailed description in case 1).
- The central partial thickness marginal tear was left to heal by secondary intention.
- Half the dosage of RIG (20 IU/kg) was injected locally around the wound and the other half intramuscularly at distant site (deltoid).

1.3.2.3 Anti-rabies Injection

Refer Table 1.2.

1.3.2.4 Discussion

Canine bites constitute the majority of the periocular animal bite injuries [8]. Rare instances of injuries caused by birds [9], bobcats [10], and human bite [11] have been reported. Children, mostly boys, between the age group 5 and 8 years are the most likely victims of familiar canine attacks and older children and adults by unfamiliar dogs [8]. There is injury to facial nerve, lacrimal drainage system particularly the canaliculi, lacrimal gland, and levator aponeurosis in dog bites [8].

A history of provoked or unprovoked attack should be elicited in victims of animal attack. Details of immunosuppressed state, diabetes, any other diseased states, prior tetanus immunization status, rabies vaccination status should be elicited [12].

Table 1.2 Post-Exposure Prophylaxis (PEP) for rabies vaccine cell-culture or embryonated egg-based vaccine for rabies PEP

Route	Regimen	Schedule
Intramuscular (deltoid muscle)	5-dose	Day 0, 3, 7, 14, 28
	4-dose	Day 0- two doses (one each in right and left arm) One dose each on day 7, day 21
	Alternate PEP in wound care +RIG[a]	Day 0, 3, 7, 14
Intradermal (i.d)	Two-site method[b]	Day 0, 3, 7, 28

[a] Alternative post-exposure regimen for healthy, fully immunocompetent exposed people who receive wound care plus high-quality rabies immunoglobulin plus WHO-prequalified rabies vaccines

[b] One i.d. injection at two sites. The volume per intradermal injection should be 0.1 mL with both purified Vero cell rabies vaccine, and purified chick embryo rabies vaccine

Examine and assess for eyelid lacerations, canalicular injury, medial and lateral canthal injuries [12]. Trauma to globe is rare but nevertheless to be looked for. In addition to the periocular region, careful examination of any facial injuries should be performed. This should be followed by a thorough copious irrigation of the wound and debridement of non-viable tissue, in the operating room if the wound is extensive. Approximately 100–200 mL of normal saline solution per inch of wound is recommended [12]. Irrigation and debridement is known to reduce the infective load of the wound by up to 90% [8, 12]. The risk of transmission of rabies can be reduced by half by washing with soap and water [7]. The timing of wound closure is controvertial [12]. Primary closure of facial and periocular wounds have better functional and cosmetic outcome with lesser chances of infection [12].

Staphylococcus, Streptococcus, and Pasteurella species are the most common organisms among others in animal bites, systemic antibiotic therapy is initiated to cover these [12]. Suggested antibiotic duration for prophylaxis is 3–5 days, 7–14 days in soft tissue infection and >3 weeks in bone involvement [8]. Amoxicillin-clavulanate is the gold standard, azithromycin in pregnant ladies or age <12 years; third-generation fluoroquinolones, trimethoprim-sulfamethoxazole, clindamycin in case of penicillin allergy [8]. Tetanus and rabies prophylaxis is recommended for all animal bite wounds [12]. The post-exposure prophylaxis (PEP) for rabies should be provided for category II and category III exposure as per WHO guidelines [13]. Category II exposure includes nibbling of uncovered skin, minor scratched or abrasions without bleeding [13]. Single or multiple transdermal bites or scratches, licks on broken skin, contamination of mucous membrane with saliva is categorized under III [13]. The PEP schedule is given in Table 1.2. In addition to vaccine, passive immunization with rabies immunoglobulin (RIG) at a dose of 20 IU/kg of human RIG is recommended for facial and periocular Category III exposure; half the dose locally injected at bite site and the other half injected intramuscularly at a distant site [13].

1.3.2.5 Conclusion

Animal bite injuries warrant an early repair, good irrigation, antibiotic coverage and anti-rabies vaccine, and RIG. Injuries involving the canaliculus should be repaired early for good outcome (Fig. 1.3c).

1.3.3 Case 3

1.3.3.1 Case Summary

A 50-year-old male presented to the eye emergency with an alleged history of road traffic accident 1 day back. He suffered trauma to face, bleeding from nose and right eyelid. There was no loss of consciousness or vomiting.

Examination revealed a complex right eyelid laceration with avulsion of the lower eyelid, bare wound at the lateral canthal area, an overhanging avulsed portion of the lower eyelid (Fig. 1.4a). The lower canaliculus was involved in laceration. He also had partial thickness laceration of the lip and philtrum. The globes were intact with an unremarkable slit lamp examination.

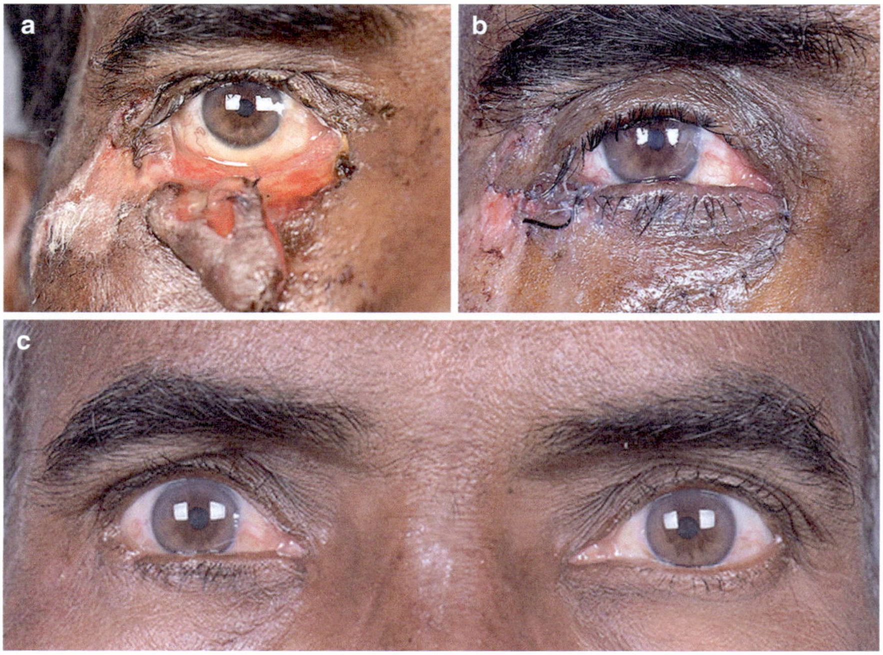

Fig. 1.4 (**a**) Clinical photograph showing complex eyelid laceration with avulsion of the lower eyelid, bare wound at the lateral canthal area, an overhanging avulsed portion of the lower eyelid involving the lower canaliculus; (**b**) immediate post-operative photo showing repaired lower eyelid; (**c**) post-operative appearance at 6 weeks

1.3.3.2 Case Management

- This was a complex eyelid laceration involving the canaliculus. Repair was performed under general anesthesia.
- After careful saline and betadine irrigation, the individual sections of the avulsed eyelid were aligned. No tissue loss was noted in the lower eyelid. Bare area lateral to lateral canthus was noted involving the superficial tissues.
- The proximal and distal ends of lacerated lower canaliculus were identified.
- The avulsed lower lid portion was anchored to the medial edge of laceration with a single 6-0 vicryl interrupted suture to aid in good approximation and ensuring tension-free repair.
- Canalicular repair was performed under microscope with mini-Monoka stent.
- Vertical mattress sutures with 6-0 silk were placed at margins, aligning the lateral end of the avulsed eyelid.
- Layered closure was performed with 6-0 vicryl interrupted sutures.
- At the lateral canthal area, edges were undermined to bring the ends closer for tension-free closure. Layered closure was performed with 6-0 vicryl interrupted sutures.
- The laceration of the lip and philtrum was repaired.

Conclusion

Complex laceration with avulsion may appear to have caused tissue loss. Careful evaluation and alignment on the operating table often reveals no tissue loss. In cases with tissue loss, advancement of wound edges by undermining, lateral canthotomy, and cantholysis can aid in good approximation of laceration edges and a neat repair.

1.3.4 Case 4

1.3.4.1 Case Summary

A 65-year-old gentleman presented to the emergency room with bleeding from his left periocular region. He allegedly had a fall from the two wheeler that he was riding and suffered an injury to the left upper face. His attender had placed a cloth with pressure on the region. The cloth was soaked with blood. After the fall, there was no loss of consciousness, no bleeding from the nose or ear, no vomiting as per the attender. On examination in the ophthalmic emergency room, his vitals were stable. He was conscious, oriented to time, place, and person. He had suffered abrasions over his left elbow and knee.

1.3.4.2 Case Management

Examination

After ensuring stable vital signs, i.e., pulse, BP, the pressure pack was gently removed from the left upper face to assess the injury. Grossly, there was a large laceration on the left brow and avulsion of the lower eyelid with periocular ecchymosis (Fig. 1.5a). Bleeding was noted from the brow laceration. A pressure pack was placed over the brow and the eye was examined. Visual acuity in the left eye was 6/12 and 6/9 in the right eye. Apart from subconjunctival hemorrhage, the examination was unremarkable in the left eye. The right eye was within normal limits.

1.3.4.3 Steps of Surgery

- Patient was planned for left eyelid and brow laceration repair under monitored anesthesia. On the operating table, the pressure pack was gently removed. The bleeding had stopped.
- Local infiltration was given and a thorough saline and betadine irrigation was done.
- On exploration under operating loupe, several glass pieces (Fig. 1.5c) were noted in the brow laceration and removed. The laceration extended up to the frontal bone (Fig. 1.5b). Frontal bone was noted to be intact.
- There was bleeding from the damaged supra-orbital vein. Hemostasis was achieved by cauterization.
- Sand particles and brow cilia were seen in the deeper tissues in the laceration that were removed and a thorough betadine was given.
- After ensuring that all the foreign bodies were removed, the edges of the brow laceration were approximated in a fashion to ensure the continuity of the brow.

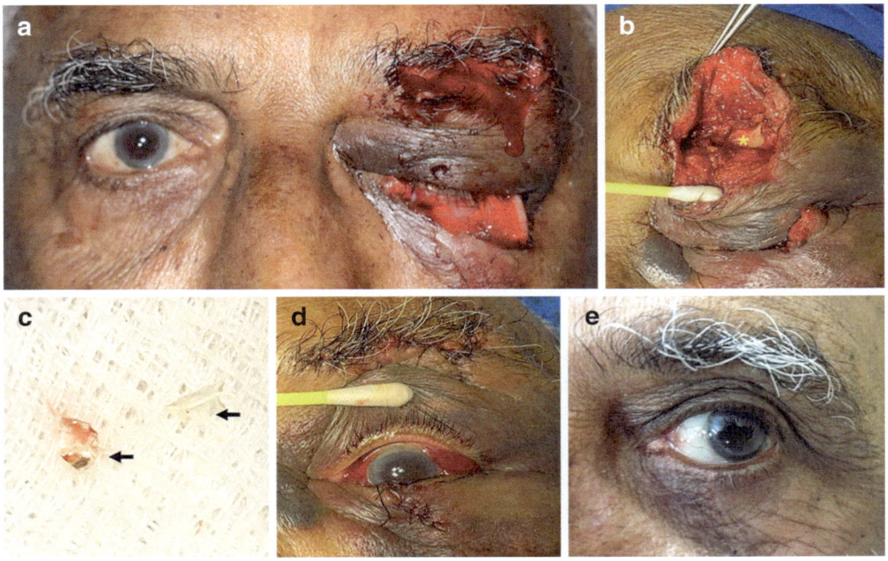

Fig. 1.5 (**a**) Full thickness laceration of the left brow and avulsion of the lower eyelid sparing the lower canaliculus; (**b**) intra-operative photograph showing the depth of the brow laceration up to the frontal bone; (**c**) glass pieces removed from the laceration during exploration before repair; (**d**) On-table appearance after completion of brow and lower eyelid repair; (**e**) Appearance after 6 months of surgery

- Layer-by-layer closure was performed. Anchoring of the ragged edges was done first with interrupted sutures. The deeper tissues were sutured with 5-0 vicryl, reverse cutting simple interrupted sutures for better tensile strength.
- The skin was closed with 6-0 vicryl interrupted sutures.
- The lower eyelid was assessed next. There was no injury to the canaliculus and no tissue loss.
- The avulsed eyelid was placed back in position and layered closure performed similar to the steps explained in previous cases (Fig.1.5d).

1.3.4.4 Surgical Pearls

- Ensure tension free approximation to minimize scarring.
- Good edge to edge approximation, minimizing tissue loss can ensure minimal scarring and reduce loss of brow cilia (Fig.1.5e).

1.3.4.5 Conclusion

- In cases of road traffic accident, look for impacted foreign bodies in the laceration wound. In case of difficulty in assessment during the initial examination in the emergency room due to bleeding, achieve hemostasis with pressure bandage and re-assess on the operating table.
- In upper eyelid and brow laceration cases, brow laceration repair is recommended before eyelid repair for better cosmesis.
- Good tension-free edge to edge wound approximation minimizes post-operative scarring.

1.3.5 Case 5

1.3.5.1 Case Summary

A 19-year-old male presented to the Oculoplasty clinic with a history of trauma to left eye with a branch of a shrub while gardening about a week ago. He suffered a tear in the lower eyelid with the branch. Upon consulting locally, a small piece of branch protruding from the wound was removed and laceration in the lower eyelid sutured. He then developed swelling around the eye, inability to move the left eye and decreased vision in the last 4 days.

The patient presented to the Oculoplasty clinic 1 week after trauma. Visual acuity was denying perception of light 8/10 times. On examination, sutured left lower eyelid laceration was noted with surrounding swelling and pus discharge (Fig.1.6a). There was severe ptosis, protrusion with chemosis, frozen left globe, and dilated fixed pupil. Fundus showed tortuous vessels. The right eye visual acuity was 6/6 with examination within normal limits.

1.3.5.2 Case Management

Computed tomography of the orbit was requested which showed a hypodense cylindrical structure (foreign body) in the infero-temporal quadrant below the inferior rectus, hematoma at the orbital apex (Fig. 1.6b). Patient was planned for exploration

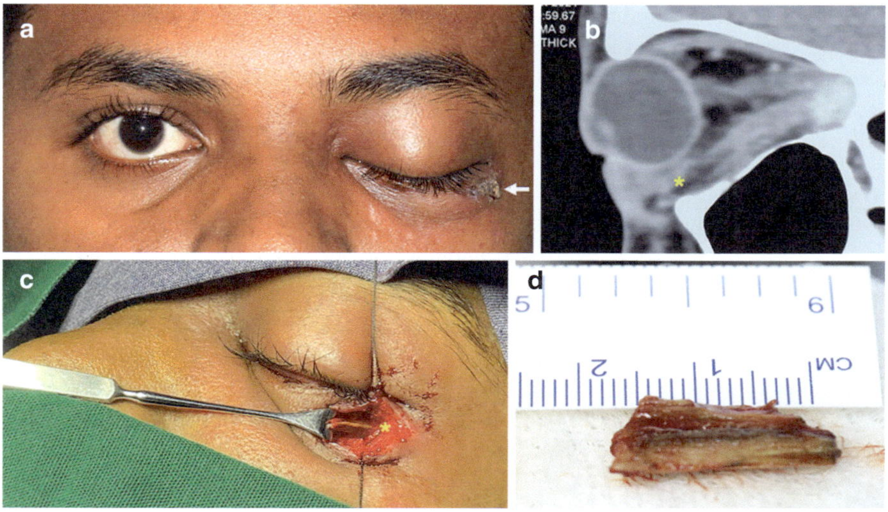

Fig. 1.6 (**a**) Repaired lower eyelid laceration with surrounding cellulitis and pus discharge; (**b**) computed tomography scan of left orbit in sagittal section showing a cylindrical hypodense structure (asterix) below the inferior rectus extending up to the middle third of orbit and hematoma at the apex; (**c**) intra-operative photograph showing the wood foreign body removed through the original lower eyelid laceration; (**d**) the piece of impacted wood removed from the left orbital apex after orbitotomy and re-exploration

and FB removal under GA. The sutured laceration site was re-opened, pus discharge was sent for microbiological examination. Gentle exploration was performed. A wood piece measuring 1.2 cm was found and removed (Fig. 1.6c). Post-operative systemic antibiotic coverage and steroids were given for hematoma at the apex.

There was some relief for the patient but the frozen globe persisted. After 1 week, repeat imaging was requested which revealed a foreign body lodged at the orbital apex. Left orbitotomy and re-exploration was performed via the original eyelid laceration and a 2 cm wood piece was removed (Fig. 1.6d).

1.3.5.3 Discussion

Cases 4 and 5 illustrate that periocular lacerations can be associated with foreign bodies (FB). A laceration, however small may seem in the initial examination, might have actually served as an entry point for a large foreign body [14, 15]. Depending on the mode of injury, foreign bodies may be lodged superficial in the wound or in the deeper tissues. Superficial foreign bodies like gravel, soil, sand, glass particles, etc. can be removed with irrigation. In injuries due to penetrating trauma, it is preferable to request pre-operative imaging like computed tomography (CT) or magnetic resonance imaging (MRI). Penetrating or deeply lodged foreign bodies should be removed in the operating room [16]. Metallic and glass FB are usually inert but nevertheless warrant removal if close to vital structures. Retained small metallic FB apart from copper can be left alone if they do not cause any functional disturbances.

Retained organic foreign bodies like wood are prone to infection and are a challenge to diagnose on CT imaging as they are difficult to differentiate from fat or air due to similar densities. MRI is preferable when suspecting organic foreign body [15, 17]. Retained organic foreign bodies can cause cellulitis, chronic inflammation, orbital abscess, fistula, and even osteomyelitis warranting early removal [17].

1.3.5.4 Conclusion

- This case highlights the importance of a thorough clinical examination and orbital imaging in the setting of penetrating trauma to rule out impacted orbital foreign body. The entry wound may be small in the periocular region, the foreign body may also look superficial on initial examination and easily removable but the suspicion of impacted orbital foreign body should be high. The direction of the entry wound gives an indication.
- It is difficult to detect wooden foreign body on imaging, serial imaging over a few days in case of high suspicion aids.

References

1. Leach J. Proper handling of soft tissue in the acute phase. Facial Plast Surg. 2001;17:227–38.
2. Hollander JE, Richman PB, Werblud M, Miller T, Huggler J, Singer AJ. Irrigation in facial and scalp lacerations: does it alter outcome? Ann Emerg Med. 1998;31:73–7.
3. Key SJ, Thomas DW, Shepherd JP. The management of soft tissue facial wounds. Br J Oral Maxillofac Surg. 1995;33:76–85.
4. Crecelius C. Soft tissue trauma. Atlas Oral Maxillofac Surg Clin North Am. 2013;21:49–60.
5. Rhee P, Nunley MK, Demetriades D, Velmahos G, Doucet JJ. Tetanus and trauma: a review and recommendations. J Trauma. 2005;58:1082–8.
6. https://www.cdc.gov/tetanus/clinicians.html#wound-management
7. Bastidas N, Levine JP, Stile FL. The "sweet science" of reducing periorbital lacerations in mixed martial arts. Ann Plast Surg. 2012;68:43–5.
8. Erickson BP, Feng PW, Liao SD, Modi YS, Ko AC, Lee WW. Dog bite injuries of the eye and ocular adnexa. Orbit. 2019;38:43–50.
9. Chaudhry IA, Al-Sharif AM, Hamdi M. Severe ocular and periocular injuries caused by an ostrich. Ophthalmic Plast Reconstr Surg. 2003;19:246–7.
10. Holzer MP, Solomon KD. Bobcat bite injury of the eye and ocular adnexa. Arch Ophthalmol. 2003;121:918–9.
11. Aguirre Vila-Coro A, Bonafonte S, Fernandez del Cotero JN. Ocular human bite. Ann Ophthalmol. 1989;21:100–2.
12. Aziz H, Rhee P, Pandit V, Tang A, Gries L, Joseph B. The current concepts in management of animal (dog, cat, snake, scorpion) and human bite wounds. J Trauma Acute Care Surg. 2015;78:641–8.
13. https://www.who.int/ith/vaccines/rabies/en/
14. Naik MN, Das S, Oluyemi F, Honavar SG. An extraordinary orbital foreign body. Ophthalmic Plast Reconstr Surg. 2011;27:e149–52.
15. Lakshmanan A, Bala S, Belfer KF. Intraorbital organic foreign body—a diagnostic challenge. Orbit. 2008;27:131–3.
16. Beadles KA, Lessner AM. Management of traumatic eyelid lacerations. Semin Ophthalmol. 1994;9:145–51.
17. Nasr AM, Haik BG, Fleming JC, Al-Hussain HM, Karcioglu ZA. Penetrating orbital injury with organic foreign bodies. Ophthalmology. 1999;106:523–32.

2 Canalicular Injuries

Manjula Sharma, Manpreet Kaur, Aditi Mehta,
and Manpreet Singh

2.1 Introduction

Canaliculi are the mucosal tubes lined by non-keratinizing squamous epithelium, located in the lacrimal portion of upper and lower eyelids. Lacrimal canaliculi connect the punctum to the lacrimal sac and play a vital role in draining tears from the lacus lacrimalis to the lacrimal sac by the lacrimal pump mechanism. Any trauma which detaches the eyelid from its strong medial canthal tendon attachments can lacerate the canaliculi. Injury in the medial canthal region affects the tear drainage system by compromising the lacrimal drainage pathway (anatomically) and the lacrimal pump function (physiologically). If not managed appropriately, it may lead to persistent clear-fluid epiphora. Hence, it becomes essential for the operating surgeon to understand the complex anatomy of this area while repairing a canalicular laceration.

The punctum is a superficial opening that draws tears from the lacus lacrimalis into the canaliculus. In 90–98% of the population, the upper and lower canaliculus joins to form a common canaliculus (length 3–5 mm) (Fig. 2.1). The lacrimal portion of the eyelids is anatomically different from the palpebral portion, as the eyelid margin is round, without eyelashes, and the absence of a tarsal plate makes it vulnerable to the traumatic avulsion.

Canalicular trauma is best evaluated by an ophthalmic surgeon experienced in the repair of canalicular lacerations. The eyelid injuries which are inadequately managed can lead to post-operative complications like eyelid margin notching,

M. Sharma
Sri Guru Harkrishan Sahib Hospital, Sohana, Mohali, Punjab, India

M. Kaur · A. Mehta
Grewal Eye Institute, Chandigarh, India

M. Singh (✉)
Department of Ophthalmology, Post Graduate Institute of Medical Education and Research, Chandigarh, India

A. Gupta, P. Tahiliani (eds.), *Oculoplastic and Orbit Casebook*, Current Practices in Ophthalmology, https://doi.org/10.1007/978-981-97-0593-1_2

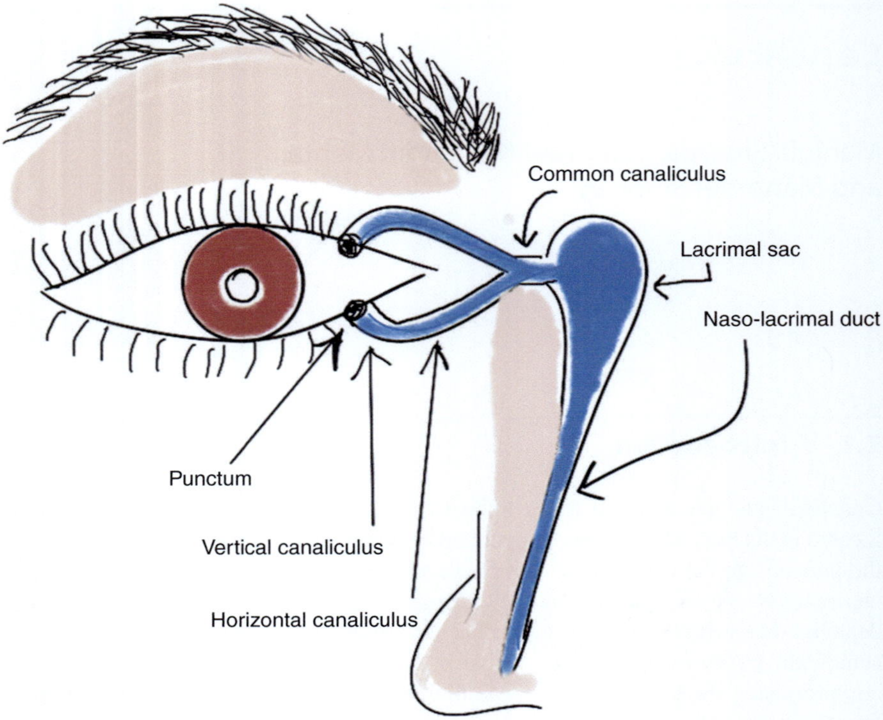

Fig. 2.1 Anatomy of lacrimal drainage system

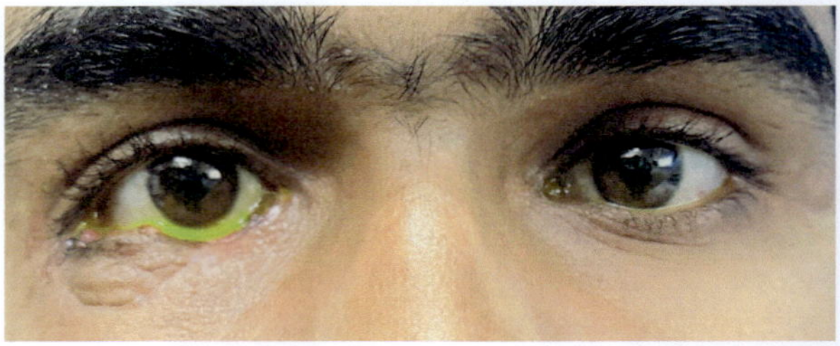

Fig. 2.2 Inadequate eyelid laceration repair leading to eyelid notching, ectropion, and persistent epiphora

lagophthalmos, traumatic ptosis, epiphora, hypertrophic scars, and wound granuloma formation [1] (Fig. 2.2).

2.2 Mechanism of Injury

Canalicular lacerations are present in approximately 16% of all eyelid injuries [2]. Wulc et al. divided canalicular lacerations based on the mechanism of injury into *direct trauma* with sharp objects (knife, glass, metal, organic material, dog bite

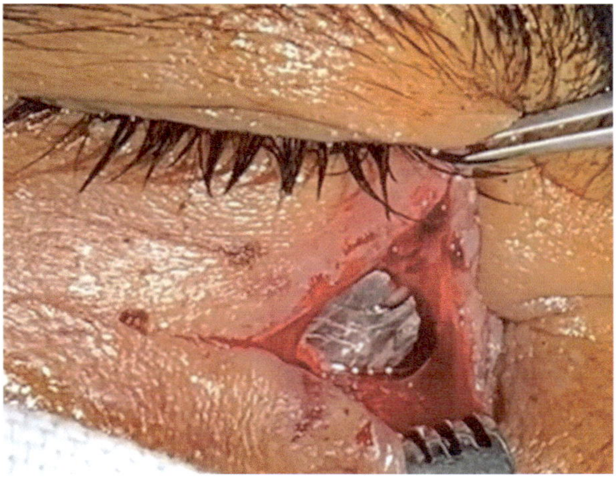

Fig. 2.3 A metallic foreign body found on wound exploration

injuries) and *indirect trauma,* such as blunt trauma (e.g., with an assault on the face, motor vehicle accident or a fall) [3].

2.3 Recording a Case History

A detailed history in a case of eyelid trauma is essential to guide the required investigations, decide the management plan, and for complete documentation of medico-legal cases in assault or road traffic accidents. Knowing the **mode of injury** will provide the information regarding the severity of injury, for example, deep lacerations and retained foreign bodies can be present in glass injuries or organic matter injury; road traffic accidents and assault can point towards associated head injury, orbital wall, or facial fractures. History regarding the *duration of injury* is also important as it can affect the prognosis and consequent morbidity.

A suspected globe perforation retained intra-orbital or intra-ocular foreign body or orbital wall fractures on history and clinical examination mandates a CT scan of the orbits (Figs. 2.3 and 2.4). Radiological scanning can help in ruling out any such trauma which, if present, may require combined surgical repair by a team of the facial plastic surgeon, ENT surgeon, and oculoplastic surgeon. MRI is contraindicated as a preliminary investigation as there can be a metallic foreign body which may lead to further inadvertent secondary trauma. A few vital points in history are:

- Tetanus immunization status.
- Animal bite (provoked, non-provoked injury) [4].
- Any history of ophthalmic, nasolacrimal surgery, facial fracture repair surgery.

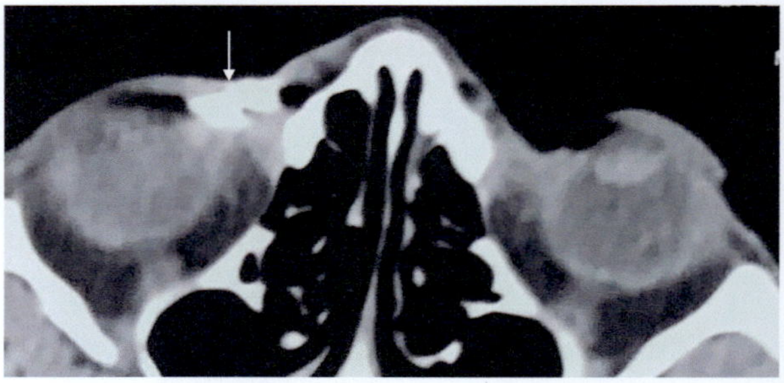

Fig. 2.4 CT scan of the orbits of the patient in Fig. 2.2 showing hyper density suggestive of a metallic foreign body

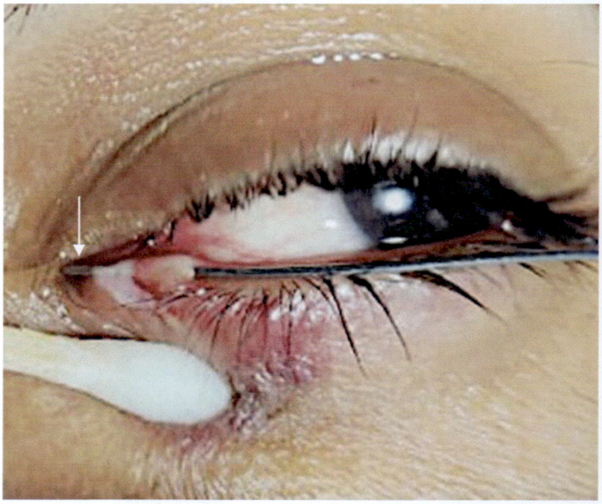

Fig. 2.5 Bowman's probe visible through the lacerated end (white arrow) of the lower canaliculus confirming canalicular injury

2.4 Examination

A canalicular laceration may not be evident on presentation due to the complex 3D anatomy of this area. It should be suspected in the following situations:

1. Any eyelid laceration medial to punctum.
2. Post-traumatic telecanthus.
3. Blunt trauma to the upper face (eyebrow, nose, cheek, lateral canthus).
4. Dog bites, glass injury.
5. Road traffic accidents affecting the face.

Examination of the eyelid laceration is preceded by copious irrigation and cleaning of the wound to remove any foreign bodies, clotted blood, and dirt particles. Canalicular injuries are identified by direct visualization of the medial eyelid, possibly under an overhead light, slit-lamp, or an operating microscope. In some cases, punctum dilatation and probing with a bowman probe may be required to confirm the findings. A visible probe within the soft tissue laceration confirms the presence of lacrimal canaliculus injury (Fig. 2.5). In children, an examination under general anesthesia may be required to confirm the diagnosis and simultaneously manage it.

2.5 Management

Repair of the eyelid margin and canaliculus is vital to restore the anatomy and function of the lacrimal drainage pathway and lacrimal pump. Multiple factors like mode of injury, the distance of laceration from punctum, type of stent used, and skill of the operating surgeon affect the outcomes of the surgery [5, 6]. As promoted by a few authors, an emergency repair within 6 h of injury is not always necessary for the best possible outcomes. Various studies have reported comparable surgical outcomes of repair within 4–5 days of injury [7–9].

Pre-operative treatment with an intramuscular tetanus booster injection (tetanus toxoid 0.5 mL) and rabies vaccination prophylaxis (in case of a dog bite) should be considered based on the patient's history. Intravenous or oral broad-spectrum antibiotic prophylaxis is recommended in infected wounds. Once the patient is stable and other associated injuries have been ruled out, it can be taken up for surgery with proper informed consent. General anesthesia is required in the case of children and adults with complex lacerations. Simple lacerations can be repaired under local anesthesia. Field blocks should be preferred rather than direct infiltration in the injured area. It is better done under an operating microscope to avoid the struggle of finding the distal end of the canaliculus and prolong surgery time. A number of techniques have been developed to repair the canaliculi

1. Direct canalicular wall anastomosis with 7-0 or 8-0 polyglactin sutures.
2. Monocanalicular stent directly or with the use of a pigtail probe (for single canalicular injuries).
3. Bicanalicular stent—looped over a prolene suture or passed into the nasal cavity (preferred in bicanalicular lacerations).
4. Monocanalicular stent into each lacerated canaliculus—in bicanalicular injuries.

Canalicular repair using a monocanalicular mini-monoka stent is an effective and most commonly preferred technique.

Instruments required for canalicular repair (Fig. 2.6):

1. Needle holder.
2. Westcott scissors.
3. Toothed forceps.
4. Punctum dilator.
5. Bowman's probe.
6. Irrigation cannula.
7. Viscoelastic/fluoresceine strips/methylene blue dye.
8. Pigtail probe-blunt tip eyed (Fig. 2.7).
9. Monocanalicular (mini-monoka stent- Fig. 2.8)/bicanalicular stent (Fig. 2.9).
10. Sutures: 5-0 prolene, 6-0 vicryl, 4-0 silk.

The intra-operative challenge is *to find the distal end of the lacerated canaliculus* as during exploration; canthal tendon fibers can mimic the cut edge of the canaliculus

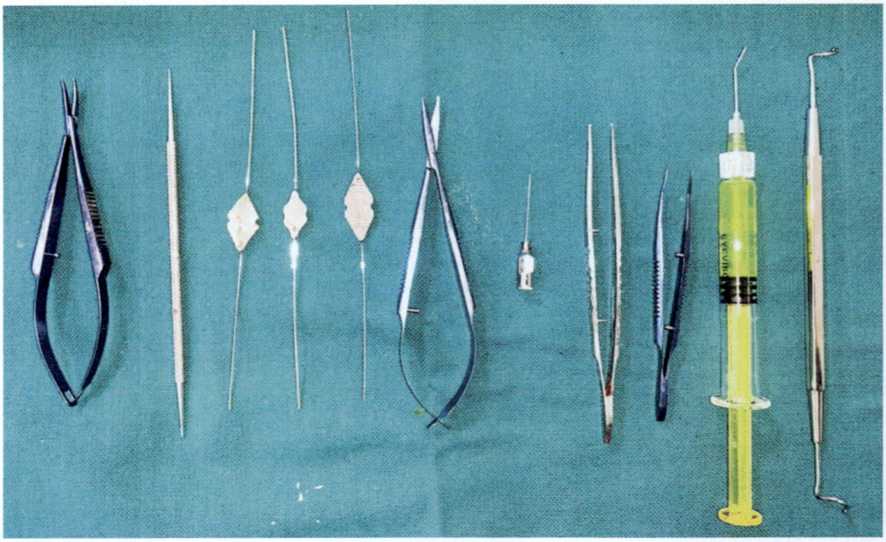

Fig. 2.6 Instruments required for canalicular repair (needle holder, punctum dilator, Bowman's probe, Westcott scissors, irrigation cannula, toothed forceps, fluoresceine-stained viscoelastic, pigtail probe)

Fig. 2.7 Blunt tip eyed pigtail probe (eye to thread the prolene suture or monocanalicular stent)

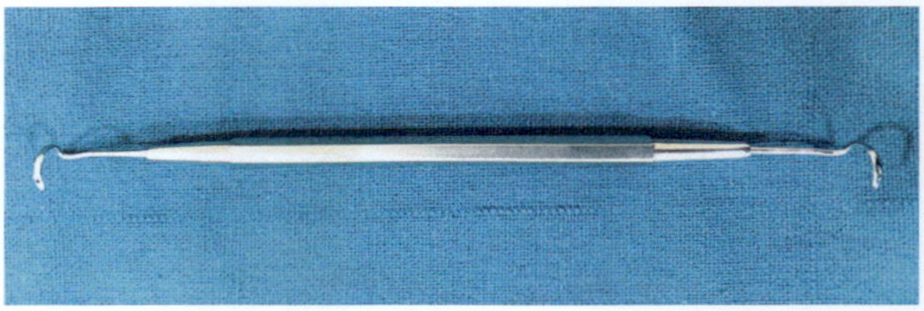

Fig. 2.8 Monocanalicular stent with the proximal punctal fixation device (white circle)

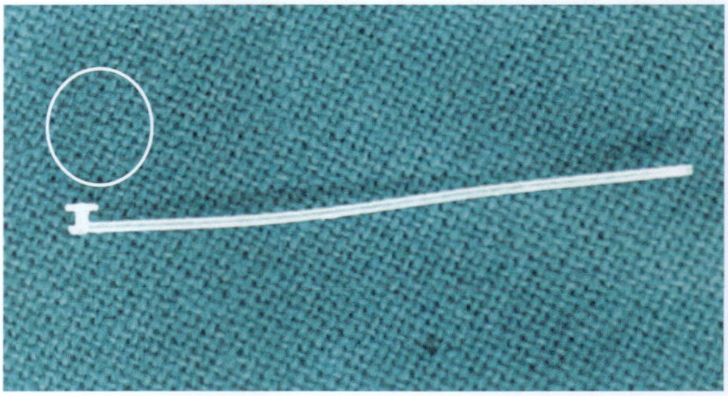

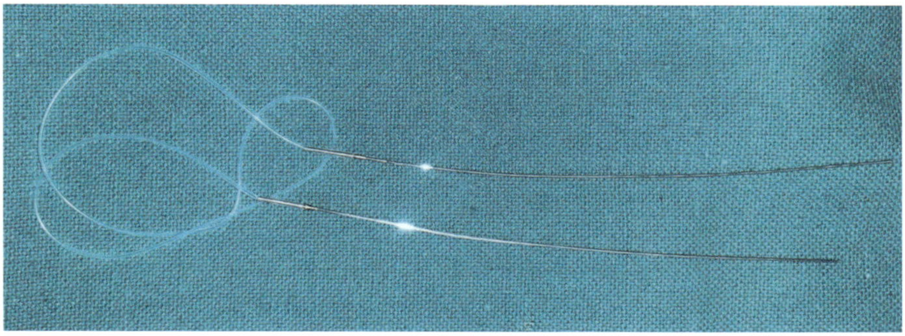

Fig. 2.9 Bicanalicular silicone stent with metallic rods to retrieve through the nasal cavity (silicone tubing has a lumen)

and edema of the surrounding tissue can make it even more challenging to identify this delicate structure. Over the years, various techniques have been developed to the locate the distal end, such as direct observation or topical phenylephrine assistance (cause constriction of the blood vessels and muscle tissues around the canaliculus) for *calamari ring sign* (whitish circular opening of the canaliculus), injecting fluoresceine stained viscoelastic, methylene blue dye or air from the opposite punctum and simultaneously seeing the appearance of viscoelastic or dye or bubbles from the distal end. In desperate cases, a blunt-eyed pigtail probe can be used in locating the distal end in patients with deeper single canalicular injuries. The authors believe that the direct magnified visualization under an operating microscope is the best way to identify the medial cut end of the lacrimal canaliculus.

2.6 Monocanalicular Laceration Repair Using Mini-Monoka Stent

(a) Closure over a monocanalicular stent: The eyelid is held with toothed forceps for stabilization, and the puncta are dilated using a punctum dilator. The stent is cut in a beveled fashion up to a length of 10 mm approximately. A mini-monoka stent is inserted into the punctum of the injured canaliculus, and the tip is retrieved from the proximal lacerated end and pulled so that its collar sits flush with the punctal ampulla. The distal end of the injured canaliculus is located using one of the above-described methods, and a stent is inserted. Pericanalicular sutures are placed using 6-0 vicryl. Conjunctiva is closed using 8-0 vicryl. Eyelid margin and eyelid are repaired using 4-0 silk.

(b) Using pigtail probe: In case of deep lacerations, a pigtail probe is required to locate the nasal end. Both puncta are dilated. A mini-monoka stent is inserted from the punctum of the injured canaliculus without trimming the length; the only tip is beveled. A pigtail probe is passed along the canaliculus from the opposite punctum, and its tip appears from the lacerated distal end of the canaliculus (Fig. 2.10). The beveled tip of the stent is threaded into the eye of the

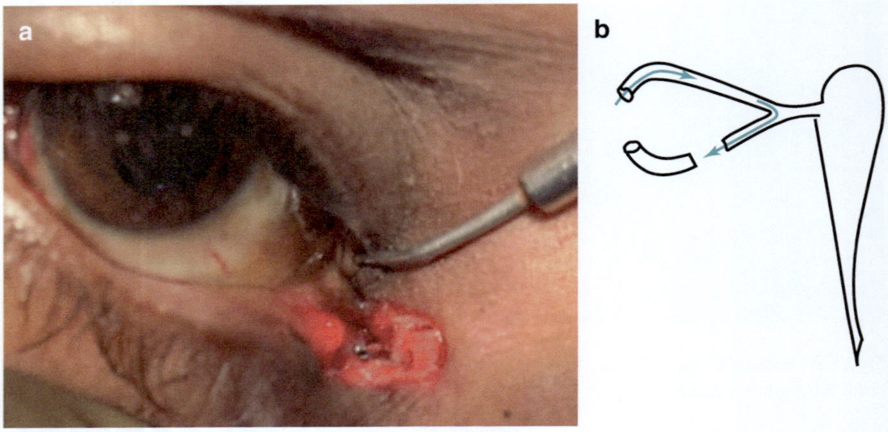

Fig. 2.10 (**a**)Pigtail probe inserted from upper punctum and blunt eyed tip visible from the distal lacerated end of lower canaliculus. (**b**) Diagramatic representation of the direction of insertion of pigtail probe

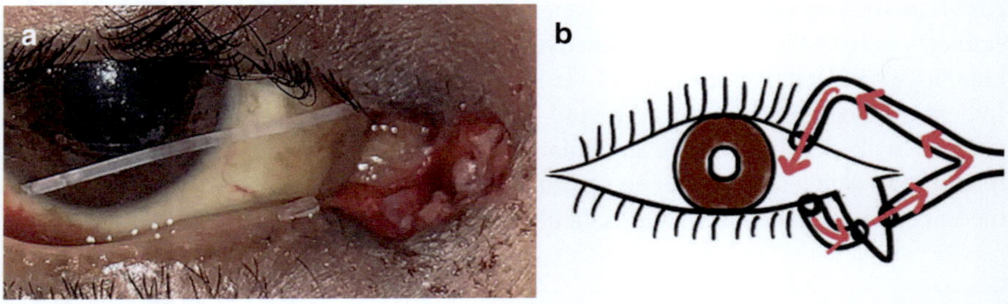

Fig. 2.11 (**a**) Monocanalicular stent is inserted from the punctum of the injured canaliculus and tip is taken out from the opposite punctum with the help of pigtail probe. (**b**) Diagramatic representation of direction of insertion of stent

pigtail probe, and the probe is retrieved back in a circular fashion so that the tip of the stent comes out from the opposite punctum (Fig. 2.11). After intubating the canaliculus, the eyelid wound is repaired as already described. The excess length of the stent protruding out from the opposite punctum can now be trimmed, or it can be secured with a single knot in the stent and vicryl suture.

2.7 Canalicular Repair Using Bicanalicular Stent

Both puncta are dilated. A pigtail probe is passed from the normal lacrimal passage, and after gently rotating it along the canaliculus, it appears from the distal injured end of the opposite canaliculus. 5-0 prolene suture is threaded into the eye of the pigtail probe, and the probe is taken out from the punctum along with the suture by rotating back. Similarly, the pigtail is passed from the punctum of the injured lacrimal canaliculus, and prolene from the distal end is threaded into the eye of the probe and taken out from the punctum. Now the prolene suture is passing from both the upper and lower canaliculus. The silicone tubing of the bicanalicular stent is trimmed to a length of approximately 25 mm. The tubing should have a lumen. Trimmed silicone tubing is passed over the already passed prolene sutures. Prolene is secured by tying the two ends, and the knot is buried into the lumen of the silicone stent. The two ends of the stent are joined by pushing one end into the lumen of the other end.

2.8 Post-op Care and Follow-up

Post-op treatment includes NSAIDS with serratiopeptidase, topical antibiotic-steroids eye drops and lubricants to prevent irritation due to stent. The patient is followed up 1 week after surgery. Eyelid margin sutures are removed 10–14 days after surgery, and stents are removed 6 weeks after surgery. Post stent removal fluoresceine dye disappearance test is done to confirm the success of the repair. Additionally, orbicularis strengthening exercises can be advised, if required, to promote the lacrimal pump mechanism.

2.9 Complications

The benefits of canalicular repair outweigh the risk of complications. There can be complications such as scarring, cicatricial ectropion, eyelid notching, stent extrusion and subsequent canalicular obstruction, punctal cheese wiring, and granuloma formation.

References

1. Nelson CC. Management of eyelid trauma. Aust NZ J Ophthalmol. 1991;19(4):357–63.
2. Herzum H, Holle P, Hintschich C. Eyelid injuries: epidemiological aspects. Ophthalmology. 2001;98(11):1079–82.
3. Wulc AE, Arterberry JF. The pathogenesis of canalicular laceration. Ophthalmology. 1991;98:1243–9.
4. Sadiq MA, Corkin F, Mantagos IS. Eyelid lacerations due to dog bite in children. J Ophthalmol Strabismus. 2015;9:1–4.
5. Singh M, Gautam N, Ahir N, Kaur M. Is the distance from punctum a factor in the anatomical and functional success of canalicular laceration repairs? Indian J Ophthalmol. 2017;65(11):1114–9.
6. Singh S, Ganguly A, Hardas A, Tripathy D, Rath S. Canalicular lacerations: factors predicting outcome at a tertiary eye care centre. Orbit. 2017;36(1):13–8.
7. Drnovsek-Olup B, Belram M. Trauma of the lacrimal drainage system: retrospective study of 32 patients. Croat Med J. 2004;45(3):292–4.
8. Chowdhury HR, Rose GE, Ezra DG. Long-term outcomes of monocanalicular repair of canalicular lacerations. Ophthalmology. 2014;121(8):1665–6.
9. Dortzbach RK, Angrist RA. Silicone intubation for lacerated lacrimal canaliculi. Ophthalmic Surg. 1985;1:185–90.

Eyelid Ptosis

3

Rwituja Thomas and Summy Bhatnagar

3.1 Case 1: Simple Congenital Ptosis

3.1.1 Introduction

Congenital ptosis is the drooping of the upper eyelid present since birth or first year of life. The ptosis can be simple or complex depending upon associated ocular or systemic involvement. Though the incidence is not well documented, *Griepentrog* et al. in their study found that approximately 81% of congenital ptosis was the simple congenital type with only 4% having bilateral involvement [1]. The ptosis is mainly a result of abnormal muscle development and can have a neurological component although this has not been elucidated clearly.

3.1.2 Case Presentation

A 22-year-old girl presented to our clinic with complaints of a droopy left upper lid since early childhood. She had no associated difficulties and was concerned about her cosmetic appearance. On examination, she had mild left eye ptosis (2 mm) with a well-defined lid fold and a margin crease distance of 6 mm in the right eye and 9 mm in the left eye (Fig. 3.1a). The ptotic left eyelid appeared higher on down-gaze as compared to the right. The phenylephrine test was negative, and ocular motility was found to be normal with no jaw-winking noted.

R. Thomas (✉) · S. Bhatnagar
Department of Orbit, Oculoplasty and Oculofacial Aesthetics, Vision Eye Centres, New Delhi, India

A. Gupta, P. Tahiliani (eds.), *Oculoplastic and Orbit Casebook*, Current Practices in Ophthalmology, https://doi.org/10.1007/978-981-97-0593-1_3

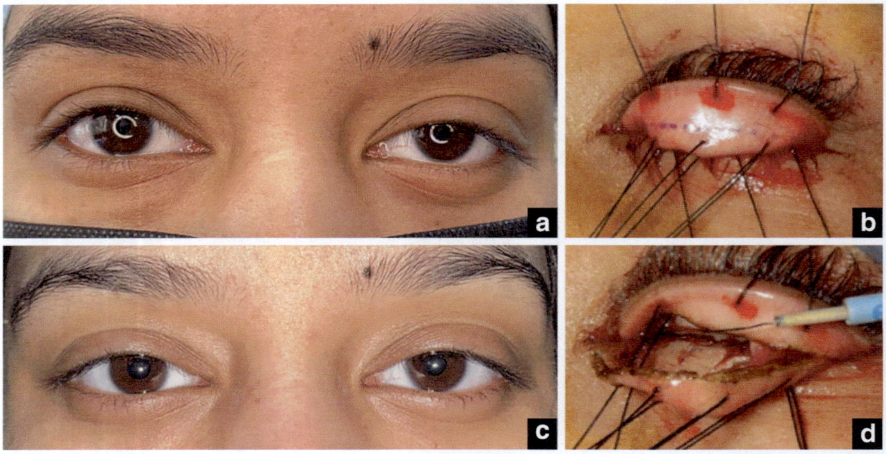

Fig. 3.1 (**a**) Left eye congenital ptosis (**b**) intraoperative marking of the incision on the folded tarsus (**c**) 6-week postoperatively (**d**) excision of the tarsus along with conjunctiva and Müller's muscle

3.1.3 Case Management

A modified Fasanella-Servat procedure was performed for our patient in her left eye. The marking was carried out based on the rule that for every 1 mm of ptosis, 2 mm has to be resected (Fig. 3.1b). Hence, the marking was made at 4 mm on the folded tarsus from the upper border of the tarsus to ensure 8 mm of tarso-conjunctivo-Müllerectomy (Fig. 3.1d). At 6 weeks postoperative, she had a symmetric lid height and contour (Fig. 3.1c).

3.1.4 Discussion

Congenital ptosis not only requires early diagnosis but appropriate and timely management as well. Varying grades of ptosis may result in astigmatism and result in refractive or deprivation amblyopia in severe cases. The drooping of eyelids affects the child physically as well as psychologically due to the cosmetic impairment. The management of ptosis mainly takes into consideration the grade of ptosis, levator muscle excursion, position of skin crease and Bell's phenomenon. The most common procedures performed are frontalis sling, levator resection (involving the Whitnall's ligament or a supramaximal one in severe cases), and the Fasanella-Servat procedure.

3.1.5 Conclusion

Among the myriad available techniques, it is the grade of ptosis, levator action, and risk of patient developing amblyopia with the other preoperative considerations that helps the surgeon with his/her experience to decide the choice of the procedure.

3.2 Case 2: Aponeurotic Ptosis

3.2.1 Introduction

Involutional ptosis also known as aponeurotic ptosis is the most common cause of acquired ptosis which presents late in adulthood. It is a result of separated levator aponeurosis and tarsus due to aging [2]. The decreased tone and thinning leads to age-related ptosis in these patients.

3.2.2 Case Presentation

A 52-year-old lady presented to us with progressive drooping of the right upper lid since the past 3 years. On examination, she had a good lid fold, higher lid crease, and a slightly deepened superior sulcus with a levator action of 13 mm on the right side. She had 1.5 mm of ptosis on the right side. The left eye had a levator action of 16 mm. On performing a phenylephrine test, a positive result was noted on the right (Fig. 3.2).

3.2.3 Case Management

This patient underwent a Müller's muscle conjunctival resection (MMCR) based on the phenylephrine test findings. A total of 8 mm of Müller's muscle was resected and sutured with an 8-0 nylon suture that was removed after 10 days. Two months after the procedure, she had an improved lid height and contour that better matched her left eye.

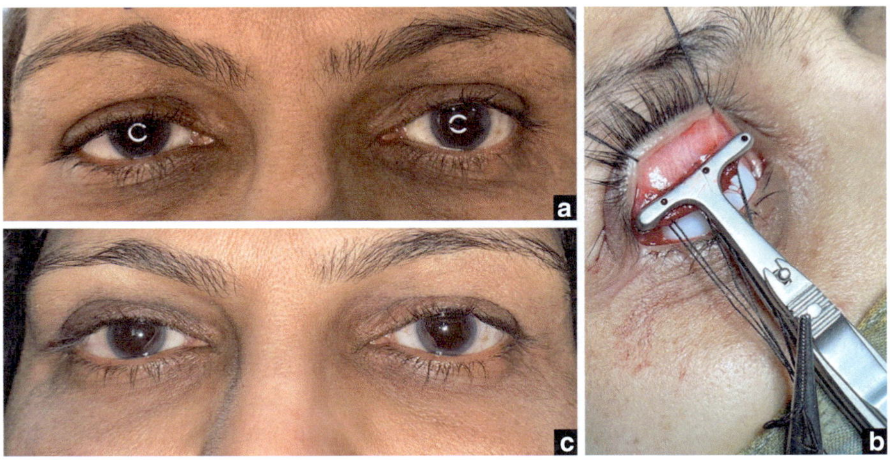

Fig. 3.2 (**a**) Right eye aponeurotic ptosis (**b**) intraoperative image of the Putterman's clamp applied on the folded conjunctiva and Müller's muscle just below the tarsus (**c**) 8 weeks postoperatively, the patient has a good lid height and contour

3.2.4 Discussion

Aponeurotic ptosis is mainly a result of aging and can be bilateral. Surgery can be performed in these cases for functional as well as cosmetic reasons. Most patients undergo levator resection for this condition and complications include undercorrection, overcorrection, and asymmetric lid fold, all of which may require surgical revision. Thus, when feasible, performing an MMCR procedure gives more predictable results; however, it is applicable only to patients with a ptosis of 2 mm or less.

3.2.5 Conclusion

Aponeurotic ptosis should be differentiated from ptosis caused by trauma or iatrogenic causes. The ptosis is usually mild to moderate. It is helpful to keep the patient on oral steroids following a levator resection, in case readjustment is needed. Achieving symmetry is the main goal of this surgery, and it takes several years and cases to master this technique. MMCR is the procedure of choice in milder cases.

3.3 Case 3: Marcus-Gunn Jaw-Winking (MGJW) Ptosis

3.3.1 Introduction

The phenomenon of Marcus-Gunn jaw-winking first was described by Robert Marcus-Gunn in 1883 [3]. It is also known as trigemino-oculomotor synkinesis or pterygoid-levator synkinesis, and on average it has been reported in 2–13% of patients who have congenital ptosis [4]. It presents with synkinetic movements of the upper eyelid on masticating movements of the mandible. It is generally has a unilateral presentation, but can rarely present bilaterally [5]. This condition affects males and females in equal proportion [6]. The synkinetic movements result from a congenital aberrant connection between the motor branches of the trigeminal nerve that control the muscles of mastication and the superior division of the oculomotor nerve that controls the levator palpebrae superioris. It can also be acquired, as in post-trauma, post-Bell's palsy, post-surgical, and due to pontine tumors [7]. Spontaneous remissions may be seen rarely in certain acquired cases.

3.3.2 Case Summary with Presentation

A 5-year-old boy presented to us with drooping of the right upper eyelid since birth (Fig. 3.3a). Ptosis was noted to cover the visual axis and the absence of lid fold was noted. On mouth opening, it was noted that there was moderate (2–5 mm) upward excursion of the right upper lid (Fig. 3.3b). The palpebral fissure height was 5 mm in the right eye (MRD1 = 0) and 9 mm in the left eye (MRD1 = 4). The levator function was 4 mm in the right and 12 mm in the left eye.

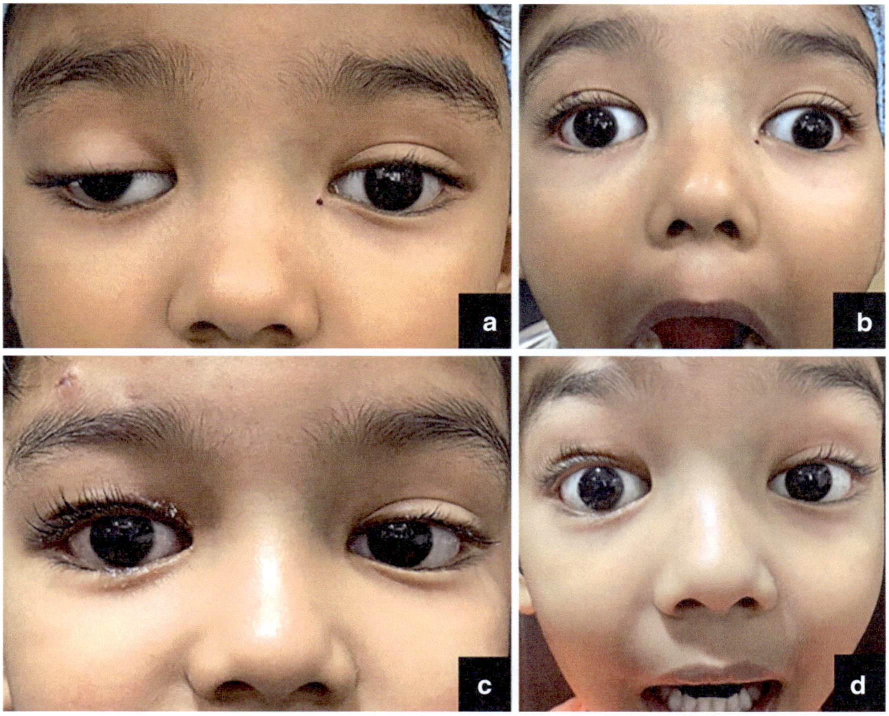

Fig. 3.3 (**a**) Right eye congenital ptosis (**b**) elevation of right upper lid on mouth opening demonstrating Marcus-Gunn jaw-winking phenomenon (**c**) 1-week post-correction of ptosis with levator excision and silastic sling in right eye (**d**) Demonstration of abolished Marcus-Gunn jaw-winking after 15 months

3.3.3 Case Images

See Fig. 3.3.

3.3.4 Case Management

After confirming the presence of a good Bell's phenomenon, a frontalis sling surgery with a silicone rod and sleeve and levator excision (short of the Whitnall's ligament) along with 2 mm width skin excision was performed. One week after the procedure, the sutures were removed, and a good lid height and contour was achieved (Fig. 3.3c) with abolished jaw-winking (Fig. 3.3d).

3.3.5 Short Discussion

The management of MGJW ptosis can be divided into medical and surgical. It is important to address vision and refraction if the ptosis is amblyogenic once correction has been achieved.

3.3.6 Surgical Care

Surgical correction in MGJW must include elimination of the synkinesis, as failure to do so can result in worsening of the abnormal eyelid movement, which may be cosmetically disfiguring. Indications for surgery include the presence of amblyopia, severe ptosis with moderate to poor levator muscle dysfunction and severe ptosis with good levator function. The jaw-winking component is considered cosmetically significant if it is more than 2 mm. Contraindications for surgery include a poor Bell's phenomenon, reduced or absent corneal sensations, and a history of or findings suggestive of dry eye disease. In our case, we did a resection of LPS with frontalis sling suspension. The procedure is a commonly followed surgical technique with better results in both synkinesis elimination and bilateral symmetry [3]. In our patient, we performed a disinsertion of LPS with frontalis sling suspension. The procedure is a commonly followed surgical technique with good results in both synkinesis elimination and obtainment of bilateral symmetry.

3.3.7 Conclusion

In the differential diagnosis of patients with ptosis, Marcus-Gunn jaw-winking syndrome should be considered and ruled out, especially if it improves during feeding, sucking, chewing, smiling, or any kind of oral movements. In case of congenital or acquired ptosis, one must always look for MGJW. The patients should be treated further on the basis of degree of ptosis and severity of jaw-winking.

3.4 Case 4: Blepharophimosis

3.4.1 Introduction

*B*lepharophimosis, *p*tosis, and *e*picanthus inversus *s*yndrome (BPES) is an abnormality of the eyelids comprising blepharophimosis, ptosis, epicanthus inversus, and telecanthus (increased intercanthal distance) present since birth [8]. BPES type I occurs in females with these four features along with primary ovarian insufficiency. BPES type II occurs without any other systemic manifestations. Other ophthalmic associations of BPES include lacrimal tract abnormalities, motility disorders, and amblyopia. Patients may additionally have craniofacial features such as a broad nasal bridge and low-set ears. It has an autosomal dominant mode of inheritance [9]. Surgery is most commonly for functional reasons, i.e., ptosis and cosmetic reasons, for correction of epicanthus and telecanthus and thus the shortened horizontal palpebral fissure.

3.4.2 Case Summary with Presentation

A 24-year-old male complained of having droopy eyelids and smaller appearance of eyes since birth. On examination, he was found to have bilateral frontalis overaction with vertical fissure height of 6 mm in both eyes. He also had horizontal shortening of the palpebral fissure and telecanthus. He also had epicanthus inversus, wherein there is a skin fold present from the lower to the upper lid medially (Fig. 3.4a). He had a poor levator function of 3 mm bilaterally with fair Bell's phenomenon.

3.4.3 Case Images

See Fig. 3.4.

3.4.4 Case Management

The surgical treatment was carried out in two stages. The first stage being a Y to V plasty which was marked (Fig. 3.4b) based on the following calculation to decide on the measurement of the long arm of the "Y":

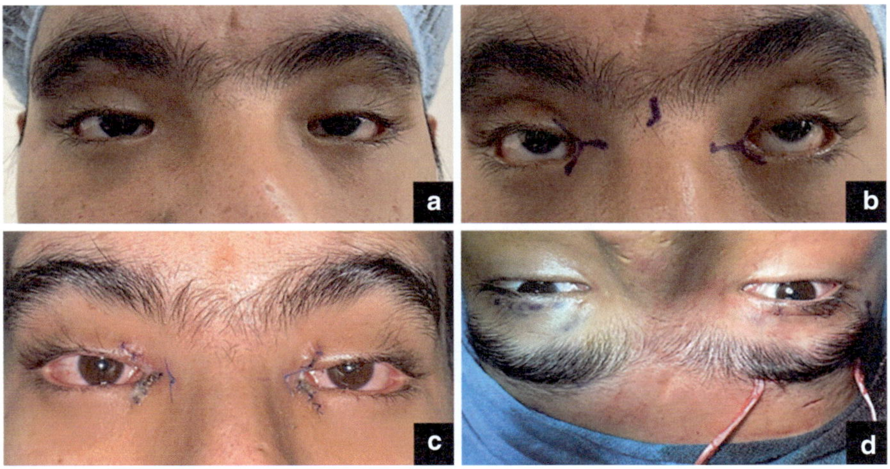

Fig. 3.4 (**a**) A patient with Blepharophimosis, telecanthus, epicanthus inversus, and bilateral ptosis (**b**) markings performed for first stage Y to V plasty based on interpupillary distance and intermedial canthal distance (**c**) 1-week post Y to V plasty with medial canthal tightening (**d**) intraoperative image of second stage surgery with fascia lata for frontalis suspension done bilaterally

Desired intercanthal distance (ICD) = Half of interpupillary distance (IPD). This was combined with the medial fixation of the medial canthal ligament onto the periosteum.

At 1 week, the intercanthal distance was at the desired level along with elongation of the horizontal palpebral fissure (Fig. 3.4c). After 12 weeks, the second-stage surgery for ptosis performed was bilateral fascia lata, with the lid fold forming on elevation with the sling (Fig. 3.4d).

3.4.5 Short Discussion

The management of this condition requires a collaborative, multidisciplinary approach with an oculoplastic surgeon, endocrinologist, and gynecologist when necessary. Ptosis surgery in these cases may be affected by dysplastic structure of the eyelids, and the aim of surgery is primary to create a cosmetically acceptable lid fold and increase the palpebral fissure height to the extent possible. Ptosis surgery is generally preceded by medial canthoplasty and Y to V plasty, double Z plasty, or C-U plasty for correction of the blepharophimosis, epicanthus inversus, and telecanthus. The ptosis correction is traditionally a bilateral fascia lata sling surgery as it provides better symmetry, especially in down-gaze in these patients. In our case also we performed a bilateral Y to V plasty followed by fascia lata sling surgery. Some surgeons have also performed supramaximal levator resection to achieve similar results [9].

3.4.6 Conclusion

BPES is not only an oculofacial abnormality, but patients may have possible endocrine manifestations along with ptosis, epicanthus inversus, and telecanthus. The eyelid surgery outcomes are satisfying both for the surgeons and the patients. Proper and timely diagnosis of the syndrome will result in best possible outcomes. Evaluation of systemic conditions should be always a part of the workup of the patients.

3.5 Case 5: Traumatic Ptosis

3.5.1 Introduction

Ptosis resulting from trauma can be due to various mechanisms, such as direct levator muscle injury, levator aponeurosis dehiscence, cicatricial bands, third nerve paresis, and combined mechanisms [10]. They can be managed by Müller-muscle conjunctival resection, levator resection or advancement, and frontalis sling surgery, based on the mechanism, response to phenylephrine test, ocular motility, and degree of levator action present.

3.5.2 Case Summary with Presentation

A 28-year-old gentleman presented to us with history of road traffic accident with head injury 3 years prior. He underwent primary repair of his open wounds and no further treatment. On examination, he was found to have severe ptosis in the right eye with the presence of a scar along the brow and glabellar region and elevated brow position (Fig. 3.5a). His Bell's phenomenon was poor with severe limitation of elevation (zero) and levator action was 0–1 mm (Fig. 3.5b).

3.5.3 Case Images

See Fig. 3.5.

3.5.4 Case Management

The patient was not a good candidate for frontalis sling surgery owing to his poor Bell's phenomenon and elevation restriction putting him at risk for exposure keratopathy if operated. Thus he was fitted with crutch glasses with a fitting incorporated on the upper part of the glasses that would temporarily lift the eyelid on wearing the glasses (Fig. 3.5c and d). This ensured cosmesis on using the apparatus as well as abolished the risk of corneal complications if surgery was performed.

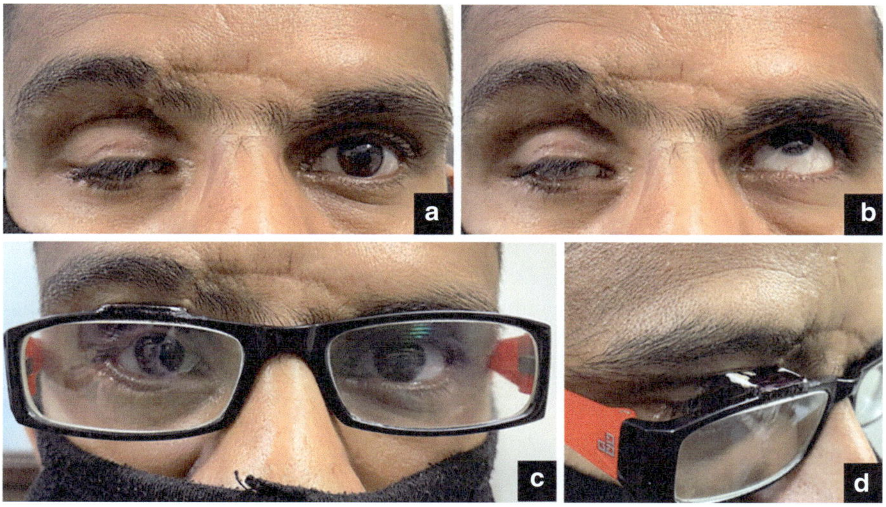

Fig. 3.5 (**a**) Right eye severe ptosis with post-traumatic scars in the glabellar and brow regions (**b**) demonstration of elevation limitation and nearly absent levator function on the right side (**c**) palpebral fissure widening in primary gaze with crutch glasses (**d**) side view of crutch glasses showing mechanical elevation of lid by crutch attachment

3.5.5 Short Discussion

Traumatic ptosis can occur following blunt or penetrating trauma, birth trauma, previous oculoplastic or strabismus surgery, or after a botulinum toxin injection in the eyelid [11]. Post trauma, a period of 3–6 months of observation is useful to look for spontaneous resolution and settling of initial inflammation. Following this, ptosis surgery can be undertaken provided it doesn't lead to any further complications such as exposure keratopathy.

3.5.6 Conclusion

In our patient, surgery was not an option due to the severely compromised ocular motility and a conservative approach was more beneficial.

3.6 Case 6: Chronic Progressive External Ophthalmoplegia (CPEO)

3.6.1 Introduction

CPEO is a mitochondrial myopathy in which young adults develop a slowly progressive ptosis and limitation in ocular motility [12]. It is a pupil sparing ophthalmoplegia. The ptosis occurs gradually and motility restriction is initially symmetric, causing the absence of diplopia. Gradually, the levator function is abolished with retention of frontalis action [13]. The ptosis in these patients is often accompanied by a poor Bell's phenomenon and dry eyes.

3.6.2 Case Summary with Presentation

A 32-year-old female presented to us with bilateral, gradually progressive drooping of eyelids and outward deviation of the eyes since the age of 16 (Fig. 3.6a). She underwent two surgeries for squint at age 22 and 26; however, the restriction of motility recurred. The patient had bilateral frontalis overaction with a palpebral fissure height of 7 mm in both eyes. She had restriction of adduction and upgaze (−4) in the left eye and restriction of upgaze (−2), abduction, and adduction (−3) in the right eye and thus a poor Bell's phenomenon in both eyes. Both eyes had normal depression.

3.6.3 Case Images

See Fig. 3.6.

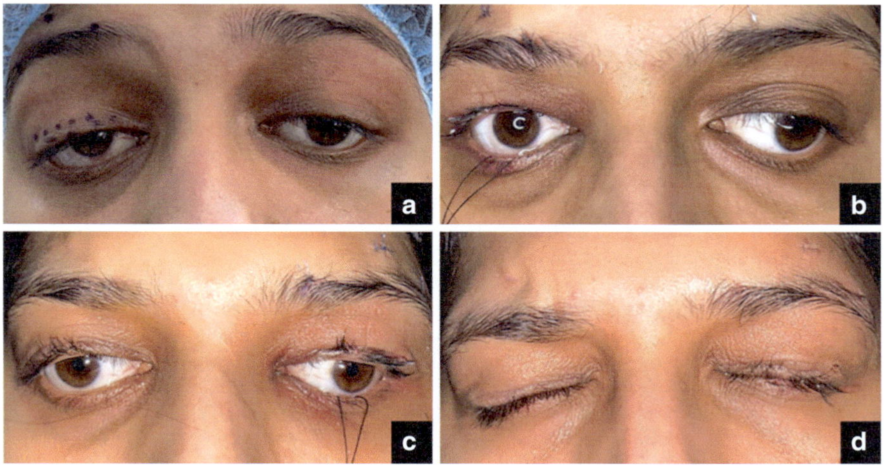

Fig. 3.6 (**a**) Demonstration of incision markings for frontalis sling with right upper lid markings for skin excision (**b**) 1-week post right eye frontalis sling suspension with good lid height, contour, and tolerance of cornea to correction (**c**) 1-week post silastic sling in left eye with good correction (**d**) No lagophthalmos

3.6.4 Case Management

We performed a frontalis silastic sling surgery in right eye (Fig. 3.6b) along with skin excision in the upper lid with a more conservative final lid height in the left eye in view of restricted upward motility. We could achieve a satisfactory outcome without any complications developing within 15 months of follow-up (Fig. 3.6c and d).

3.6.5 Discussion

As there is no medical cure for CPEO, the main management strategy is that of symptom control. When patients experience diplopia, they can be treated with prism lenses or with strabismus surgery. As the levator function is poor in the later stages of the disease, patients require frontalis sling surgery as was done in our patient, keeping in mind a conservative approach to avoid complications such as exposure keratitis. Silicone slings are a good option due to their flexible nature [13].

3.6.6 Conclusion

As CPEO is a clinical diagnosis, it is important to rule out other differentials such as myasthenia gravis and thyroid eye disease. The surgical treatment for ptosis can drastically improve the quality of life of the patients. A complete ocular examination, with focus on the myogenic and neurogenic aspects, is essential to diagnose CPEO and distinguish between its phenotypes.

References

1. Griepentrog GJ, Diehl NN, Mohney BG. Incidence and demographics of childhood ptosis. Ophthalmology. 2011;118(6):1180–3.
2. Lee YG, Son BJ, Lee KH, Lee SY, Kim CY. Clinical and demographic characteristics of blepharoptosis in Korea: a 24-year experience including 2,328 patients. Korean J Ophthalmol. 2018;32(4):249.
3. Senthilkumar VA, Tripathy K. Marcus Gunn jaw winking syndrome. In: StatPearls [Internet]. Treasure Island: StatPearls Publishing; 2022. [cited 2022 Jun 15]. Available from: http://www.ncbi.nlm.nih.gov/books/NBK559058/.
4. Doucet TW, Crawford JS. The quantification, natural course, and surgical results in 57 eyes with Marcus Gunn (jaw-winking) syndrome. Am J Ophthalmol. 1981;92(5):702–7.
5. Weaver RG, Seaton AD, Jewett T. Bilateral Marcus Gunn (jaw-winking) phenomenon occurring with CHARGE association. J Pediatr Ophthalmol Strabismus. 1997;34(5):308–9.
6. Khwarg SI, Tarbet KJ, Dortzbach RK, Lucarelli MJ. Management of moderate-to-severe Marcus-Gunn jaw-winking ptosis. Ophthalmology. 1999;106(6):1191–6.
7. Joshi M, Tailor M, Ghugare B. Trigemino-oculomotor synkinesis: report of a rare case. J Indian Acad Oral Med Radiol. 2014;26(1):92.
8. Mari F, Giachino D, Russo L, Pilia G, Ariani F, Scala E, et al. Blepharophimosis, ptosis, and epicanthus inversus syndrome: clinical and molecular analysis of a case. J AAPOS. 2006;10(3):279–80.
9. Decock CE. Increased levator muscle function by supramaximal resection in patients with blepharophimosis-ptosis–epicanthus inversus syndrome. Arch Ophthalmol. 2011;129(8):1018.
10. Jacobs S, Tyring A, Amadi A. Traumatic ptosis: evaluation of etiology, management and prognosis. J Ophthalmic Vis Res. 2018;13(4):447.
11. Boyle NS, Chang EL. Traumatic Blepharoptosis. In: Cohen AJ, Weinberg DA, editors. Evaluation and management of blepharoptosis [Internet]. New York: Springer New York; 2011. [cited 2022 Jun 15]. p. 129–40. Available from: http://link.springer.com/10.1007/978-0-387-92855-5_13.
12. Riordan-Eva P. Vaughn & Ashbury's general ophthalmology. England: Lange Medical Bks; 2007.
13. Eshaghi M, Arabi A, Eshaghi S. Surgical management of ptosis in chronic progressive external ophthalmoplegia. Eur J Ophthalmol. 2021 Jul;31(4):2064–8.

Ectropion and Entropion

4

Aditi Mehta

4.1 Introduction

Eyelid margin malposition is a frequently encountered disease entity. Ectropion refers to outward turning of the eyelid with loss of apposition to the globe. Entropion is an inward turning of the eyelid, resulting in lash-globe contact. This chapter entails description of these two diseases, the pathophysiological types, clinical evaluation and management along with a few relevant cases.

Anatomically, the eyelids are a trilamellar structure. The anterior most lamella consists of the skin, subcutaneous tissue, and orbicularis oculi muscle, which is further categorized into orbital, pre-septal, and pretarsal orbicularis. The middle lamella consists of pre-septal fat, orbital septum, and the post-septal fat pad—two in upper eyelid and three in lower eyelid. The posterior lamella consists of the tarsal plates (10 mm height in upper eyelid and approximately 5 mm height in lower eyelid), the conjunctival lining, and the eyelid retractors—Levator Palpebrae Superioris and Müller's muscle in upper eyelid and capsulopalpebral fascia in lower eyelid [1].

Kakizaki described the two layers of the lower eyelid retractors—anterior and posterior. The anterior layer is a fine capsulopalpebral expansion of the inferior oblique muscle in continuation with the Lockwood ligament. It fuses with orbital septum 4–5 mm from the inferior tarsal border and then continues through the orbicularis oculi fibers to terminate in the subcutaneous tissue of the anterior lamella, forming the lower eyelid crease. It helps stabilize the anterior lamella of the eyelid and its vector has an everting action. The posterior layer is thicker. It consists of dense connective tissue and smooth muscle fibers of the capsulopalpebral expansion of inferior rectus muscle insertion. It inserts on the lower border of tarsus. This partially muscular posterior layer retracts on detachment from the tarsus. It maintains eyelid margin position and stabilizes the tarsal plate by exerting a downward

A. Mehta (✉)
Grewal Eye Institute, Chandigarh, India

A. Gupta, P. Tahiliani (eds.), *Oculoplastic and Orbit Casebook*, Current Practices in Ophthalmology, https://doi.org/10.1007/978-981-97-0593-1_4

and backward pull, to keep it against the globe. It also plays a role in keeping the visual axis clear in downgaze by transmitted movement of inferior rectus muscle. These two layers can be separated on dissection but remain linked by interconnective tissue [2].

The eyelid margin from anterior to posterior consists of the lash line along the eyelash follicles, the gray line of muscle of Riolan (orbicularis oculi fibers), the meibomian gland orifices in the tarsal plate and the mucocutaneous junction which is the sharp border with conjunctiva.

4.2 Part I: Ectropion

4.2.1 Definition and Types

Eversion of the eyelid with loss of globe—eyelid apposition results in ectropion. The lower eyelid is more frequently involved, due to the additional effect of gravity. The various types include congenital, cicatricial, mechanical, paralytic, and involutional ectropion.

Congenital ectropion is rare and is usually associated with euryblepharon (or megaloblepharon) and blepharophimosis epicanthus inversus syndrome [3]. It is caused by vertical insufficiency of anterior lamella and may be associated with epiphora and exposure keratitis. It must be differentiated from acute eyelid eversion resulting from orbicularis spasm due to birth injury (Adam's bilateral congenital upper eyelid eversion) or due to conjunctivitis leading to anterior lamellar inflammation [4]. While congenital eyelid eversion may resolve spontaneously, eyelid laxity associated with euryblepharon requires surgical horizontal eyelid shortening. Ectropion at birth may also be seen in lamellar ichthyosis, the hallmarks of which are skin thickening and scaling.

Cicatricial ectropion is associated with traumatic pyrogenic or chemical burns, cicatrizing skin diseases, and post-trauma or post-surgical resection with eyelid tissue loss resulting in anterior lamellar shortening. Treatment is surgical—scar tissue has to be released followed by reconstruction with skin/composite grafts to replace the anterior lamella of eyelids.

Mechanical ectropion results from a lesion near the eyelid margin which pulls on the eyelid. Removal of the lesion along with eyelid reconstruction can help in resolution.

Paralytic ectropion is seen in patients of Bell's palsy (VII nerve) resulting in downward displacement of the lower eyelid due to paralysis of orbicularis oculi muscle and loss of tone. Associated findings included reduced facial animation on the affected side, upper eyelid lagophthalmos due to paralytic upper eyelid orbicularis, poor Bell's reflex and resultant exposure keratopathy. Acute cases may be managed conservatively with lubrication, eyelid taping and tarsorrhaphy; surgical correction is required in chronic cases with incomplete resolution. Medial canthoplasty for medial ectropion with or without lateral canthal elevation (lateral tarsal strip or canthal sling) for lateral ectropion are required. For generalized laxity, additional midface lift may be needed along with the horizontal tightening procedures.

Involutional ectropion is commonest and frequently affects the lower eyelid due to the anatomy as well as effects of gravity.

Pathophysiology of involutional ectropion and entropion:

- The lower eyelid is suspended like a hammock at the medial and lateral canthal tendons. The horizontal vector keeps it taut along x axis and the vertical vector forces of capsulopalpebral fascia and lower eyelid retractors provide the upward pull along y axis. This vertical force is counterbalanced by the effects of gravity which causes a downward pull. Age-related horizontal laxity leads to loss of tautness. Depending on the status of the vertical vectors—ectropion or entropion may develop.
- When the lower eyelid retractors are disinserted, their extensions to the overlying orbicularis oculi and skin also dehisce. The increased tone of pre-septal orbicularis then causes an override over the pretarsal orbicularis, rotating the eyelid margin towards the globe leading to *entropion.*
- If the lower eyelid retractors are disinserted, laxity is present along the tarsal sling at the medial and lateral canthal tendons, and the orbicularis tone is also weakened, the unopposed effect of gravity leads to the development of *ectropion*.
- The bilamellar nature of the lower eyelid retractors also explains the development of ectropion and entropion. The disinserted posterior layer with an intact anterior layer causes an external rotation of tarsus leading to ectropion. In contrast, dehiscence of both anterior and posterior layers of the lower eyelid retractors leads to entropion as orbicularis override develops producing an inverting action [2, 5].
- Upper eyelid involutional entropion develops due to horizontal and vertical laxity. The Müller's muscle and Levator Palpebrae Superioris act in the vertical upward direction, counterbalanced by downward gravitational pull. Disinsertion or weakness of these leads to blepharoptosis along with inward turning of eyelid margin; orbicularis override is usually not contributory.
- Upper eyelid involutional ectropion is less common and may be associated with floppy eyelid syndrome.

4.2.2 Examination

A thorough clinical evaluation starts with relevant history including onset of symptoms, prior ocular trauma, periorbital or ocular surgery, prior inflammatory and allergic diseases, history of facial burns, and a history of eye rubbing. Common symptoms in ectropion include inferior scleral show (in mild cases, it is usually the first sign but may remain asymptomatic), epiphora, irritation, gritty eye with foreign body sensation, mucoid discharge, lagophthalmos, and cosmetically disfiguring eyelid eversion. Another symptom which may be elicited on questioning is epiphora which gets relieved in supine position. On lying down, the lax eyelid in the absence of effect of gravity, falls back on the globe enabling punctal contact with the lacrimal lake and relieving epiphora.

Physical examination includes assessment for facial dysmorphism, midface hypoplasia leading to lower eyelid retraction, and eyelid scarring (cicatricial ectropion). Facial animation including forceful eyelid closure should be tested to evaluate orbicularis and facial muscle weakness associated with VIIth nerve palsy and lagophthalmos (paralytic ectropion). In involutional cases, along with the eyelid malposition, we may find additional changes of eyelid laxity including steatoblepharon, dermatochalasis, and involutional blepharoptosis.

Extent of eyelid involvement should be noted in order to classify the ectropion as generalized, medial or lateral. Ectropion limited to medial eyelid results in punctal eversion, loss of contact of puncta in lacus lacrimalis, and epiphora. The epiphora causes discomfort for which patients may resort to frequent eye rubbing to wipe the tears, further precipitating the eyelid laxity and worsening of ectropion. In long standing cases, punctal stenosis may also be noted due to "disuse atrophy" as the tears drain by spilling onto the eyelid skin. In such situations, syringing should be done to evaluate for proximal as well as distal blockage. Next, the eyelids should be examined for inflammation, skin discoloration, blepharitis, mass lesions, madarosis, keratinization, and palpebral conjunctival scarring. Testing for eyelid laxity is essential for clinical evaluation and planning the management especially in involutional cases. Horizontal lower eyelid laxity may be assessed by placing a thumb at the lateral canthus to push the eyelid laterally and superiorly. On this maneuver, the eyelid margin may roll back into position indicating involutional ectropion. Failure to do so may point towards conjunctival forniceal scarring and a cicatricial component. Cicatricial ectropion is also accentuated when the anterior lamella is put on maximum stretch by asking the patient to look upward while simultaneously opening his or her mouth.

Grading systems are available for lower eyelid laxity [6]. Medially, the lower eyelid is pulled laterally and the punctal position is graded from 0 to 6, corresponding to displacement in millimeters (mm). If the puncta is minimally displaced, the laxity is grade 0. If the puncta can be distracted up to the medial limbus (approximately 2 mm), the laxity is mild; up to mid pupillary plane (in primary gaze)—moderate and up to lateral limbus—severe. Lateral canthal laxity is assessed on medial traction and measured in millimeters. The eyelid distraction test (pinch test) involves pulling the lower eyelid away from the globe up to 2–3 mm is normal; ≥5 mm indicates substantial laxity. The snap back test involves downward traction onto lower eyelid and release after which the time taken to return to normal position is noted. The normal eyelid springs back spontaneously. In addition, on downward pull, a white line of dehisced retractor band may be seen. These tests are summarized in Table 4.1.

According to the Ectropion Grading Scale, the clinical severity of ectropion is as follows [7]:

- 0—Normal eyelid appearance and function
- I—Normal eyelid appearance but minimally symptomatic, laxity present on examination
- II—Scleral show without eversion of the eyelid

Table 4.1 Grading for eyelid laxity

Test	Grade 0 (normal)	Grade I	Grade II	Grade III	Grade IV
Snap back test	Returns to position immediately	2–3 s	4–5 s	>5 s	Never returns to normal position
Medial canthal laxity	0–1 mm displacement	2 mm	3 mm	>3 mm	Does not return to baseline
Lateral canthal laxity	0–2 mm	2–4 mm	4–6 mm	>6 mm	Does not return to baseline, even with blink

- III—Ectropion without eversion of the inferior lacrimal punctum
- IV—Advanced ectropion with eversion of punctum from lacrimal lake
- V—Ectropion with a complication like conjunctival metaplasia, retraction of anterior lamella, stenosis of lacrimal system
- L—Predominantly lateral ectropion
- M—Predominantly medial ectropion
- t—Previous tarsorrhaphy

4.2.3 Management

The management of ectropion depends on the extent of symptoms and causative mechanism. A useful algorithm for assessment and management of ectropion is presented below in Table 4.2.

4.2.4 Discussion with Clinical Cases

1. **Cicatricial Ectropion**: 30y/M with a history of burns injury to face and upper body including arms, 3 weeks prior (Fig. 4.1a). On evaluation, there was involvement of forehead, bilateral periorbital regions and upper, and bilateral upper and lower eyelid ectropion. After initial healing, and conservative management, the patient was reexamined at 3 months (Fig. 4.1b) to allow adequate healing for better uptake of donor skin graft. Donor area was chosen as the retroauricular region for skin graft because it was not involved in the burns' injury and the skin color and texture matches the eyelid skin. Post scar excision and ectropion release, the eyelids were reconstructed with skin graft for replacement of anterior lamella. At the 6 weeks follow-up, the donor site was well healed (Fig. 4.1c) and the ectropion was well corrected in the right eye. Residual lateral ectropion was noted in the left eye; however, there was no lagophthalmos on eyelid closure (Fig. 4.1d).

   Discussion: Cicatricial ectropion is usually secondary to burns or chemical injury and may be extensive. Scarring is prominent on examination and one should allow adequate healing of recipient bed before planning reconstruction.

Table 4.2 Management algorithm for ectropion

Type	Classification	Management options
Ectropion since birth	Congenital	• Inverting suture • Horizontal tightening for euryblepharon
Ectropion with mass lesion	Mechanical	Surgical removal of lesion and eyelid reconstruction
Ectropion with skin shortening	Cicatricial	• Z plasty for localized small scars—the middle stroke of Z is along the scar to excise it and gain vertical length • Skin graft/flap for large defects and skin loss
Ectropion with poor eyelid closure	Paralytic	Temporary measures including lubrication and tarsorrhaphy; horizontal eyelid shortening: Lateral tarsal strip or lateral canthopexy *May need to add gold weight in upper eyelid for lagophthalmos*
Ectropion with eyelid laxity	Involutional-generalized	• Bick's procedure—full thickness triangular resection of lateral eyelid • Full thickness pentagon wedge resection for eyelid laxity without canthal tendon laxity • Kuhnt Szymanowski (KS) procedure—eyelid split with tarsal wedge resection and skin excision; Smith's modification—additional blepharoplasty for dermatochalasis • Lateral tarsal strip procedure *May need to add Jone's plication for lower eyelid retractor reattachment if dehisced* *May need to add midface superficial musculoaponeurotic system (SMAS) lift for age-related periorbital changes*
	Medial	• Ziegler's cautery inferior to puncta • Medial conjunctival spindle excision and retractor plication with inverting spiral suture for punctal inversion • Medial canthal tendon plication/resection • Byron-Smith Lazy T procedure—medial full thickness wedge resection with medial conjunctival spindle excision and retractor plication, inferior to puncta *May need to add punctal snip for stenosis*
	Lateral	• Lateral tarsal strip (LTS); add upshift if associated midface (maxillary) hypoplasia • Lateral tarsal sling/canthopexy

While localized immature scars may be treated with perilesional steroid and 5-Fluorouracil injections, extensive scarring requires release and replacement of the anterior lamella (skin and orbicularis tissue). Forearm, retroauricular and supraclavicular regions are well-matched donor sites for skin grafting.

2. **Congenital Ectropion:** Fig. 4.2a: Congenital ectropion associated with BPES (blepharophimosis epicanthus inversus syndrome). The left lower eyelid is proportionately longer (euryblepharon) leading to laxity and ectropion. Figure 4.2b: Lower eyelid ectropion associated with ichthyosis. The arrows point towards the scaly skin on forehead and neck. Figure 4.2c: Child with amniotic band syndrome with left anophthalmos, bilateral lip and cleft palate, right-sided lower

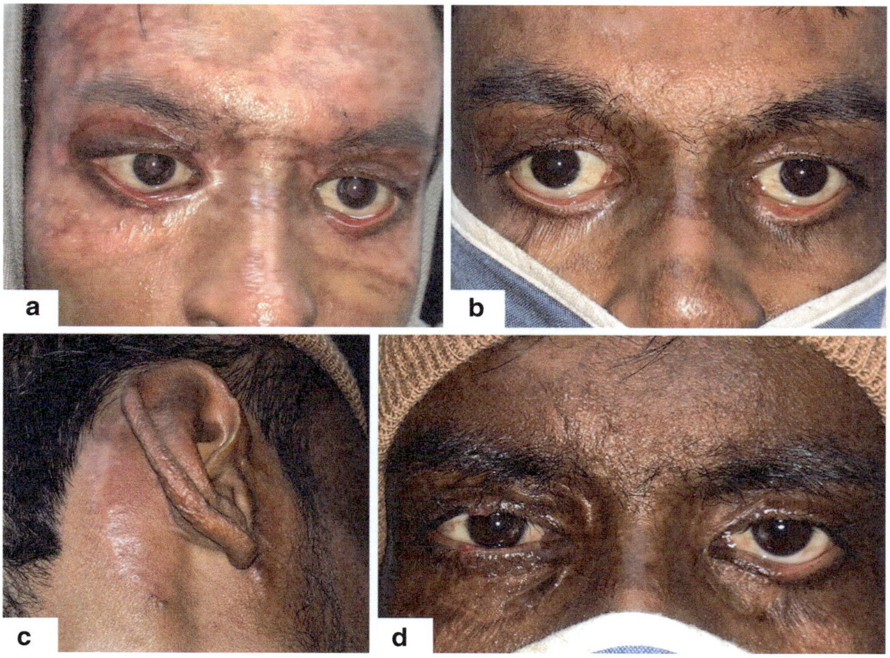

Fig. 4.1 Clinical Case of Cicatricial Ectropion: 30y/M with a history of burns injury acute presentation (**a**). After initial healing and conservative management, the patient was reexamined at 3 months (**b**). At the 6 weeks follow-up after skin grafting from retroauricular region, the donor site was well healed (**c**) and the ectropion was well corrected in the right eye. Residual lateral ectropion was noted in the left eye (**d**); however, there was no lagophthalmos on eyelid closure

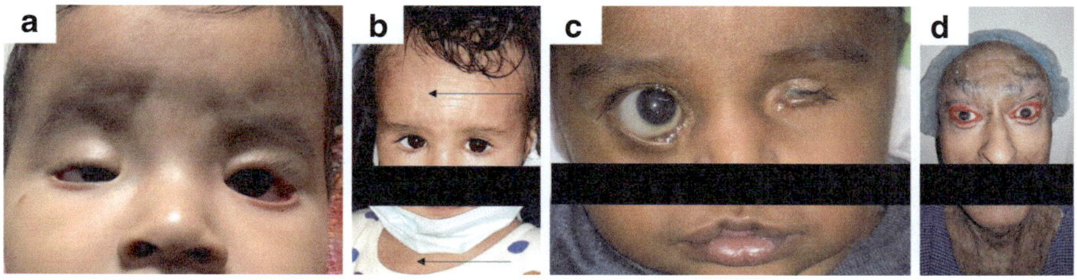

Fig. 4.2 Clinical Case of Congenital Ectropion: (**a**) Congenital ectropion associated with BPES (blepharophimosis epicanthus inversus syndrome). (**b**) Lower eyelid ectropion associated with ichthyosis. The arrows point towards the scaly skin on forehead and neck. (**c**) Child with amniotic band syndrome with left anophthalmos, bilateral lip and cleft palate, right-sided lower eyelid coloboma, and medial ectropion. (**d**) An adult patient with ichthyosis with bilateral upper and lower eyelid ectropion

eyelid coloboma and medial ectropion likely from a failure of eyelid fold fusion and associated midface hypoplasia. Figure 4.2d: an adult patient with ichthyosis with bilateral upper and lower eyelid ectropion.

Discussion: Ectropion at birth may be associated with other developmental defects (Fig. 4.2a and c) or systemic conditions like ichthyosis (Fig. 4.2b) [8]. The presentation may be dramatic as it is cosmetically disfiguring and may have associated functional defects. Thorough evaluation and systemic assessment are necessary. Treatment may be multi-staged and it is important to include conservative measures to prevent corneal exposure and keratopathy.

3. **Involutional Ectropion:** Fig. 4.3a: 65y/M with mild bilateral lower eyelid involutional ectropion. Note the outward turned eyelid margin, periorbital dermatochalasis, senile blepharoptosis, and steatoblepharon. A functional dye disappearance test was positive for epiphora while syringing was patent indicating a functional block due to eyelid laxity and associated orbicularis weakness with failure of lacrimal pump. Figure 4.3b: Severe senile (involutional ectropion) with keratinization along lateral half of left lower eyelid. Figure 4.3c: Mild ectropion involving both upper and lower eyelids in a 40y/M. Although the periorbital aging changes are not noted (and not expected at this age), the patient has history of frequent eye rubbing due to seborrheic blepharitis leading to significant eyelid laxity. The seborrheic scales are noted along the eyelashes when the eyelids are closed.

   Discussion: Involutional ectropion is seen in the aging patients and is associated with eyelid laxity; mild cases are usually asymptomatic. Examination reveals outward turned eyelid margin with visualization of the posterior eyelid margin in primary gaze and prominent eyelid laxity. Periorbital laxity is noted in the form of dermatochalasis, steatoblepharon, senile blepharoptosis, and brow ptosis. Epiphora causing constant periocular irritation and conjunctival exposure may lead to secondary keratinization in long standing cases. Premature eyelid

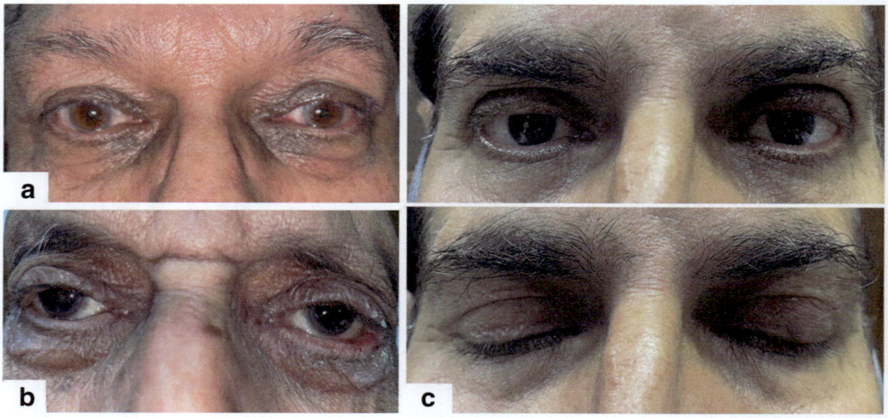

Fig. 4.3 Clinical Case of Involutional Ectropion: (**a**) 65y/M with mild bilateral lower eyelid involutional ectropion. Note the outward turned eyelid margin, periorbital dermatochalasis, senile blepharoptosis, and steatoblepharon. (**b**) Severe senile (involutional ectropion) with keratinization along lateral half of left lower eyelid. (**c**) Early onset mild ectropion in a 40y/M. Although the periorbital aging changes are not noted (and not expected at this age), the patient has history of frequent eye rubbing due to seborrheic blepharitis leading to significant eyelid laxity. The seborrheic scales are noted along the eyelashes

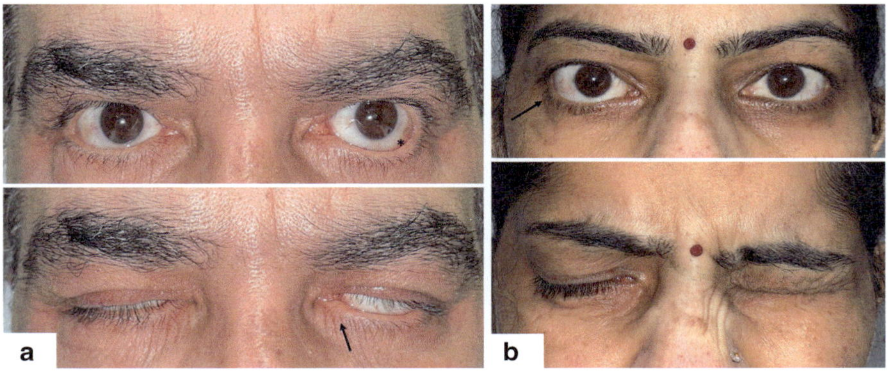

Fig. 4.4 Clinical Case of Paralytic Ectropion: (**a**) Residual paralytic ectropion after left facial nerve palsy. Inferior scleral show (asterix), lagophthalmos and predominantly medial ectropion with poor punctal apposition (arrow) is noted. (**b**) 38y/F with congenital right facial nerve palsy with lateral scleral show (arrow)

laxity may be associated with eyelid rubbing and eyelid inflammation as seen in seborrheic blepharitis. It is important to treat the underlying cause before surgical correction of ectropion.

4. **Paralytic Ectropion** Fig. 4.4a: Mild ectropion affecting the left lower eyelid. Inferior scleral show (asterix) lagophthalmos and predominantly medial ectropion with poor punctal apposition (arrow) is noted. The lazy T procedure is appropriate for the management of this case. Figure 4.4b: 38y/F with congenital facial nerve palsy with lateral scleral show in the right eye and right lower eyelid laxity. Facial animation testing with forceful eye closure depicts poor orbicularis tone on the right side. A lateral tarsal strip may lead to adequate resolution and restoration of cosmesis in this case.

   Discussion: Paralytic ectropion is seen in incompletely recovered VIIth nerve palsy patients and testing for facial animation is necessary. In patients with incomplete recovery and residual palsy, the periocular signs may be subtle and limited to inferior scleral show and lagophthalmos. In acute cases, temporary measures including lubrication and tarsorrhaphy are essential to prevent corneal exposure. Definitive surgical management of ectropion is planned after recovery for cases with incomplete resolution.

4.3 Part II: Entropion

4.3.1 Definition and Types

Malposition of the eyelids resulting in inward turning of the eyelid margin and eyelash-eyeball contact is known as entropion. Entropion can cause corneal and conjunctival injury resulting in corneal stromal abrasion, corneal neovascularization, and scarring as well as corneal thinning and ulceration in long standing cases. Like ectropion, the etiology is varied and entropion can affect both the upper and lower eyelids. The main types include congenital, cicatricial, acute spastic, and involutional.

Congenital entropion may result from tarsal kinking during birth trauma, disinsertion/dysgenesis of lower eyelid retractors or posterior lamellar vertical insufficiency. It is important to differentiate this entity from epiblepharon—wherein a horizontal fold of redundant eyelid skin and orbicularis oculi muscle along the eyelid margin cause the eyelashes to be directed vertically. Epiblepharon is more common in Asian pediatric population and may resolve spontaneously as the child grows. In contrast in entropion, the eyelid margin is also inverted and needs surgical repair. Another differential is congenital distichiasis wherein an additional row of eyelashes may arise from the meibomian gland orifices leading to eyelash-cornea contact. Treatment is indicated if keratopathy develops—lubricants may suffice initially; cryo/electro-epilation and eyelid splitting with follicle removal may be required.

Cicatricial entropion results from shortening of the posterior lamella due to inflammatory fibrosis and scarring. Associated conjunctival and ocular surface changes may be present including symblepharon, forniceal shortening, keratinization, and loss of eyelid margin architecture—all hallmarks of inflammation. Etiology may include trachoma, herpetic disease, ocular cicatricial pemphigoid, Stevens-Johnson syndrome, and other progressive inflammatory diseases.

Acute spastic entropion is an intermittent entropion resulting from spasm of the orbicularis oculi muscle leading to override of the pre-septal over the pretarsal muscle, more commonly affecting the lower eyelid. It is thought to be a precursor to persistent involutional lower eyelid entropion. The spasm is usually induced or unmasked by local irritation, infection, or recent ocular surgery. Treatment of underlying local irritation and epilation of offending eyelashes rubbing onto the cornea is required. Though it may resolve on its own, chemo-denervation of orbicularis oculi with botulinum toxin may provide temporary relief. Assessment for underlying eyelid laxity is important as involutional entropion may ensue.

Involutional entropion is the commonest type resulting from age-related eyelid laxity, disinsertion of lower eyelid retractors, and overriding of orbicularis oculi. As discussed in the pathophysiology section in part I, it is the vertical vector force which decides the direction of eyelid malposition and development of entropion. Complete lower eyelid retractor dehiscence and orbicularis override are frequently encountered in entropion [5].

- Histological examination of tarsal plates in patients with involutional eyelid entropion has shown degenerated collagen fibers and abnormal elastogenesis. These factors are responsible for increased horizontal eyelid laxity. In addition, smaller tarsal plates allow for more horizontal laxity and orbicularis override—which is why entropion is commoner in females as they have smaller tarsal plates [9].
- Orbital fat and volume decrease with age and/or after trauma resulting in relative enophthalmos. This produces an increased spacing between the globe and eyelid, leading to eyelid laxity and producing an orbicularis override. Shorter axial

length and lower measurement on Hertel exophthalmometry are known to be associated with entropion. Asian race and females are relatively enophthalmic contributing to higher rates of entropion in these populations [10].

4.3.2 Examination

Patients with entropion usually present earlier in the course of disease due to eyelashes rubbing onto the ocular surface leading to foreign body sensation, tearing, and redness. Examination for eyelid malposition begins with assessment of facial morphology. In view of the morbidity of eyelash-cornea contact, the corneal and conjunctival surface should be stained with fluorescein dye and examined under cobalt blue filter for signs of corneal abrasion, punctate keratitis, and ocular surface health. Inward directed eyelashes are also encountered in trichiasis, distichiasis, and epiblepharon which are the differentials that should be considered. In trichiasis, the eyelid position is normal, but the eyelashes are misdirected as a result of scarring, commonly seen in trachomatous eyelids. Distichiasis is a congenital disorder wherein eyelashes originate abnormally from the meibomian gland orifices along the posterior eyelid margin. Epiblepharon is seen in Asian pediatric population and results from a horizontal fold of redundant skin and orbicularis at the normally positioned eyelid margin. The eyelashes may be directed vertically or inverted inside to a small degree but signs of corneal abrasion are infrequent. In contrast, in congenital entropion, the eyelid margin is inverted.

Eyelid skin should be examined for signs of inflammation. Ocular surface should be evaluated for symblepharon, forniceal shortening, eyelid margin keratinization, and other signs of inflammation and scarring, especially in cicatricial entropion. Resistance to traction, inability to evert the eyelid, and persistence of entropion with horizontal eyelid traction can indicate cicatricial component. In contrast, involutional entropion gets corrected on horizontal eyelid traction, and eversion is easy as the eyelids are lax. In addition to entropion, eyelid retraction may be noted in cicatricial cases. When present, surgical posterior lamellar lengthening with grafts is required.

The Kemp and Collin grading of upper eyelid entropion is as follows [11]. In minimal entropion, there is apparent posterior migration of the meibomian glands with conjunctivalization of eyelid margins and eyelash contact with globe on upgaze. This can be managed with anterior lamellar repositioning (ALR) after eyelid split at the gray line. Moderate entropion includes eyelashes touching globe in primary gaze position with thickening of tarsal plate and eyelid retraction. This requires tarsal wedge resection along with ALR or transverse blepharotomy and eyelid margin rotation to redirect the eyelashes and correct the retraction due to thickened tarsus. Severe entropion results from eyelid retraction causing incomplete closure, gross eyelid distortion, presence of metaplastic eyelashes, and keratinization of eyelid margin. Surgical management includes posterior lamellar advancement via rotation of terminal tarsus or posterior lamellar graft and rotation of terminal conjunctival edge. Mucous membrane grafting may be added after removing the keratinized margins.

History and clinical evaluation for hemifacial spasm or blepharospasm is important for suspected spastic entropion as the management is with botulinum toxin rather than surgical correction. Intermittent spastic entropion may be evaluated with tests for induced entropion—TIE and TIE-2. These are indicated in cases where clinically no entropion is observed but symptoms suggest intermittency. The test of induced entropion (TIE) test involves instillation of topical anesthetic followed by instructing the patient to look in downgaze. The skin of the lower eyelid is pinched, rolled over the superior tarsal border, pressed and spread against the globe, and then released. The patient is instructed to keep looking down throughout the test. If the entropion persists with eye movements and blinking for at least 3 min, a diagnosis of spastic entropion is suspected [12].

The test of induced entropion −2 (TIE-2) is performed in three steps. After asking the patient to look down, the upper eyelid is held as high as possible by the examiner, and then the patient is instructed to close their eyes as tightly as possible. This induces the orbicularis override leading to lower eyelid entropion in patients with spastic entropion [13].

Eyelid laxity is assessed as described for ectropion. In addition to horizontal laxity, rounding of eyelid margin and retractor weakness or disinsertion is common. Lower eyelid retractor function is measured by noting the excursion of lower eyelid in downgaze; normal is 3–4 mm, and it may be reduced or absent if retractors are dehiscent. On slit lamp examination of the inferior fornix, presence of a white line 3–4 mm inferior to the lower border of tarsus indicates a disinserted retractor band. Tests for eyelid laxity are described in Fig. 4.5. A 70y/M presented with senile entropion of right lower eyelid (Fig. 4.5a). Figure 4.5b demonstrates the snap back test; the dashed line represents the white band of dehisced retractors. Figure 4.5c depicts the pinch test and Fig. 4.5d and e demonstrate testing for lateral and medial canthal laxity; the block arrows depict direction of pull.

4.3.3 Management

Management options are summarized below (Table 4.3). Some procedures aimed at correcting horizontal eyelid laxity are the same as for ectropion. The aim in entropion surgery is to achieve slight overcorrection at end of surgery as subsequently with eyelid blinking, slight inward turning of eyelid is expected.

4.3.4 Discussion with Clinical Cases

1. **Congenital Epiblepharon**: Fig. 4.6a: A 9-month-old child with apparent entropion of left lower eyelid. On examination, the eyelashes were vertically directed, but the eyelid margin was normally positioned (Fig. 4.6b). This is seen in epiblepharon.

   Discussion: Epiblepharon is an additional skin fold along lower eyelid which causes the eyelashes to be directed vertically up. It is seen in the congenital age

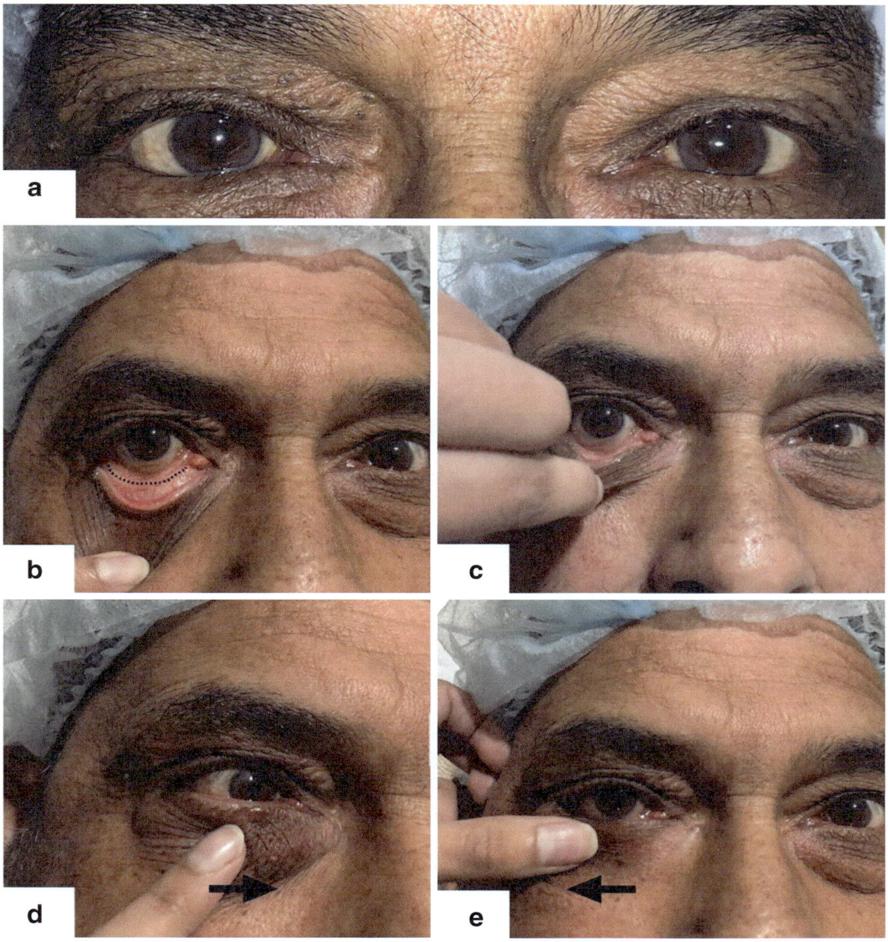

Fig. 4.5 Tests for eyelid laxity. A 70y/M presented with senile entropion of right lower eyelid (**a**). (**b**) Demonstrates the snap back test; the dashed line represents the white band of dehisced retractors. (**c**) Depicts the pinch test and (**d** and **e**) demonstrate testing for lateral and medial canthal laxity; the block arrows depict direction of pull

group and usually resolves on its own. Lubrication is required to prevent corneal erosions. Congenital entropion is rare. The eyelid margin itself is in turned and requires surgical correction.

2. **Cicatricial Entropion** (Fig. 4.7): An elderly lady presenting with bilateral upper eyelid entropion and eyelid retraction. In addition to arcus senilis, bilateral corneal pannus was noted as indicative of chronic inflammation and healed keratitis. She underwent bilateral transverse blepharotomy with eyelid margin rotation.

   Discussion: Cicatricial entropion is typically progressive and arises from inflammatory scarring leading to relative shortening of the posterior lamella

Table 4.3 Management algorithm for entropion

Type	Classification	Management options
Entropion since birth	Congenital	• Quickert Rathbun everting sutures • Hotz procedure—subciliary skin and orbicularis excision with reattachment of lower eyelid retractors to tarsal plate and overlying skin • Tarsal kink removal with margin rotation
Entropion with posterior lamella shortening	Cicatricial	• Tarsal fracture—transverse blepharotomy and margin rotation with eversion of distal tarsus if eyelid retraction is up to 1.5 mm • Hard palate/auricular cartilage graft for reconstruction of tarsal plate in severe cases with posterior lamellar deficiency • Gray line eyelid split and retractor repositioning or anterior lamellar recession to address trichiasis *Additional electro-epilation/lash follicle excision/ cryo-epilation may be required for severe trichiasis*
Entropion with orbicularis override	Spastic; involutional	• Botulinum toxin into lower eyelid • Wheeler's procedure—orbicularis transposition to prevent override • Wies procedure—everting sutures with full thickness transverse eyelid split for orbicularis override • Quickert procedure—everting sutures with full thickness eyelid split with wedge resection for associated horizontal laxity
Entropion associated with eyelid laxity	Involutional	• Quickert procedure (as above) • Jone's procedure—transverse eyelid split with wedge resection with lower eyelid retractor plication • Full thickness pentagon wedge resection for eyelid laxity without canthal tendon laxity • Kuhnt Szymanowski (KS) procedure—eyelid split with tarsal wedge resection and skin excision; Smith's modification—additional blepharoplasty for dermatochalasis • Lateral tarsal strip procedure *May need to add Jone's plication for lower eyelid retractor reattachment if dehisced in any of the above procedures*

(tarsus). The Kemp and Collin classification (described above) provides a useful management algorithm for upper eyelid entropion. In this case, there was eyelash globe contact in primary gaze with thickened tarsal plate and approximately 1.5 mm eyelid retraction, making it a moderate entropion. The patient underwent transverse blepharotomy and eyelid margin rotation with a satisfactory result.

3. **Spastic Entropion** (Fig. 4.8): Before and after injection botulinum toxin in orbicularis oculi in a case of bilateral spastic entropion. Periorbital dermatochalasis is suggestive of eyelid laxity and patient was diagnosed with combined intermittent spastic and involutional entropion.

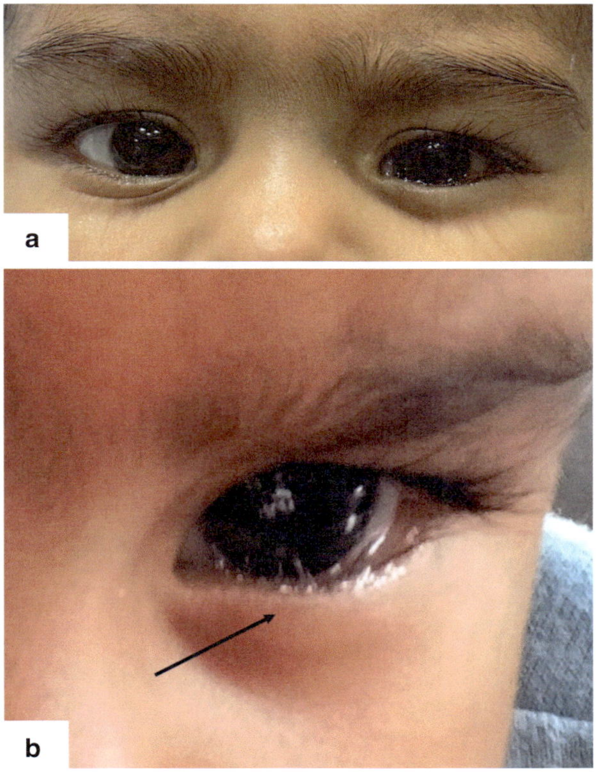

Fig. 4.6 Clinical Case of Congenital Epiblepharon: (**a**) A 9 -month-old child with apparent entropion of left lower eyelid. On examination, the eyelashes were vertically directed, but the eyelid margin was normally positioned (**b**). This is seen in epiblepharon

Discussion: Patients undergoing botulinum toxin injection for spastic entropion usually require multiple injections after the effect has worn off. However, aggressive doses can result in iatrogenic ectropion in the setting of eyelid laxity. Persistent or recurrent entropion suggests an underlying involutional entropion for which surgery is required.

4. **Involutional Entropion:** Fig. 4.9a and b: Before and after Jone's Plication and skin-orbicularis excision for right lower eyelid involutional entropion. This patient had vertical and horizontal eyelid laxity with retractor dehiscence, the canthal distraction was not significant. Figure 4.9c and d: Before and after Lateral Tarsal Strip + Jone's Plication and skin-orbicularis excision for right lower eyelid involutional entropion in view of generalized horizontal laxity including lateral canthal laxity and retractor dehiscence.

   Discussion: Involutional entropion is commonly encountered in clinics and requires surgical correction. The lateral tarsal strip surgery is a workhorse procedure for correcting eyelid laxity. Jone's plication is necessary when lower eyelid retractors are dehisced. A combination of surgeries is often required. Associated dermatochalasis may also be addressed but care has to be taken to not induce asymmetry in unilateral cases undergoing surgery.

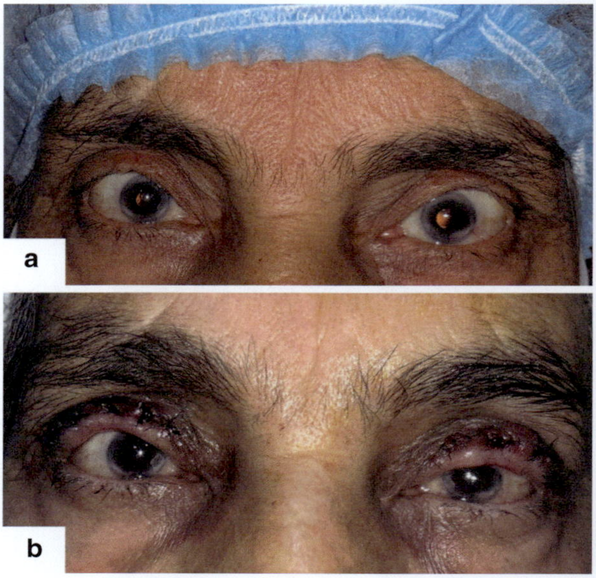

Fig. 4.7 Clinical Case of Cicatricial Entropion: An elderly lady presenting with bilateral upper eyelid entropion and eyelid retraction (**a**). In addition to arcus senilis, bilateral corneal pannus was noted indicative of chronic inflammation and healed keratitis. She underwent bilateral transverse blepharotomy with eyelid margin rotation (**b**)

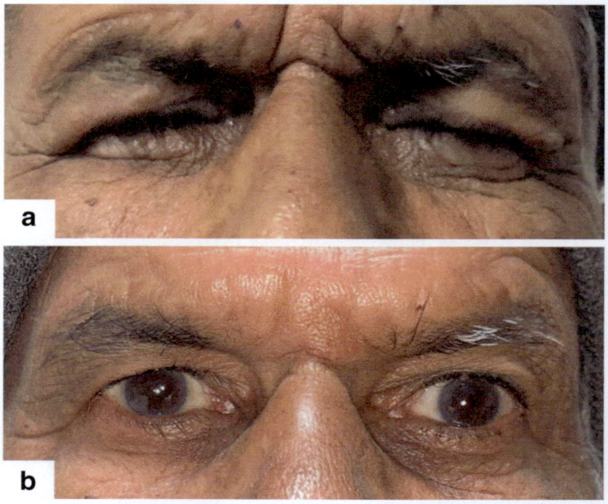

Fig. 4.8 Clinical Case of Spastic Entropion: Before (**a**) and after (**b**) injection botulinum toxin in orbicularis oculi

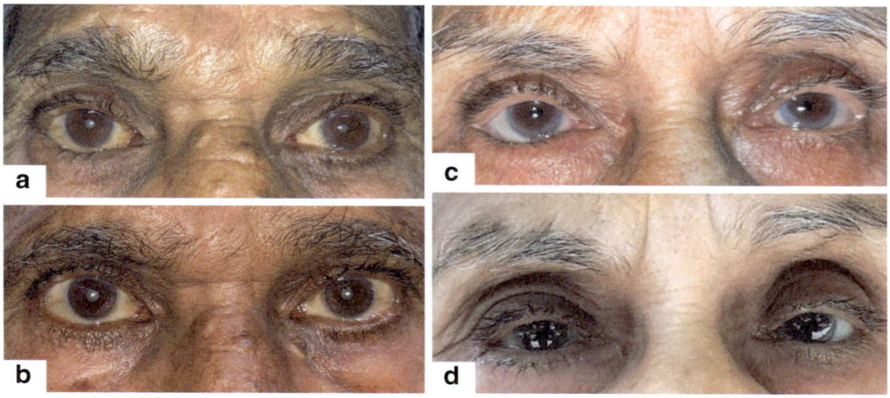

Fig. 4.9 Clinical Cases of Involutional Entropion: (**a** and **b**) Before and after Jone's Plication and skin-orbicularis excision for right lower eyelid involutional entropion. (**c** and **d**) Before and after Lateral Tarsal Strip along with Jone's Plication and skin-orbicularis excision for right lower eyelid involutional entropion

4.4 Conclusion

Eyelid malposition—ectropion and entropion are frequently encountered in the clinic. Clinical examination provides clues for etiology. Management is algorithmic and aims to relieve symptoms of epiphora (ectropion) or eyelash rubbing (entropion). Surgical correction when performed is aimed at achieving an end point of adequate correction in ectropion and slight overcorrection in entropion, especially in involutional lower eyelid malposition. Three main surgical procedures which are routinely performed include the lateral tarsal strip, Jone's lower eyelid retractor plication, and medial conjunctival spindle excision.

The lateral tarsal strip is a useful procedure for correcting horizontal eyelid laxity. The surgical steps are described briefly in Fig. 4.10. Under local anesthesia, lateral canthotomy and inferior cantholysis are performed. The eyelid margin is split at the gray line along the lateral aspect (approximately one-third, depending on the amount of horizontal laxity). The conjunctiva inferior to tarsus is incised to obtain a strip of tarsus. The conjunctiva on posterior surface of the tarsal strip is scratched off with a sharp instrument to avoid an inclusion cyst. The tarsal strip is held and pulled towards the lateral orbital rim to titrate the amount of excision required. Once excised, the remainder strip is hitched to the periosteum just inside the lateral orbital rim with a non-absorbable suture. The lateral canthus is reformed and excess skin in the gray line split anterior lamella is excised.

Jone's plication of dehisced lower eyelid retractors is essential in addressing involutional entropion and ectropion. The surgical steps are described in Fig. 4.11. Under local anesthesia, a horizontal skin incision is made approximately 4–5 mm below the eyelash line along the length of the eyelid, ending just lateral to the puncta. The orbicularis is incised along the length of the incision to expose the

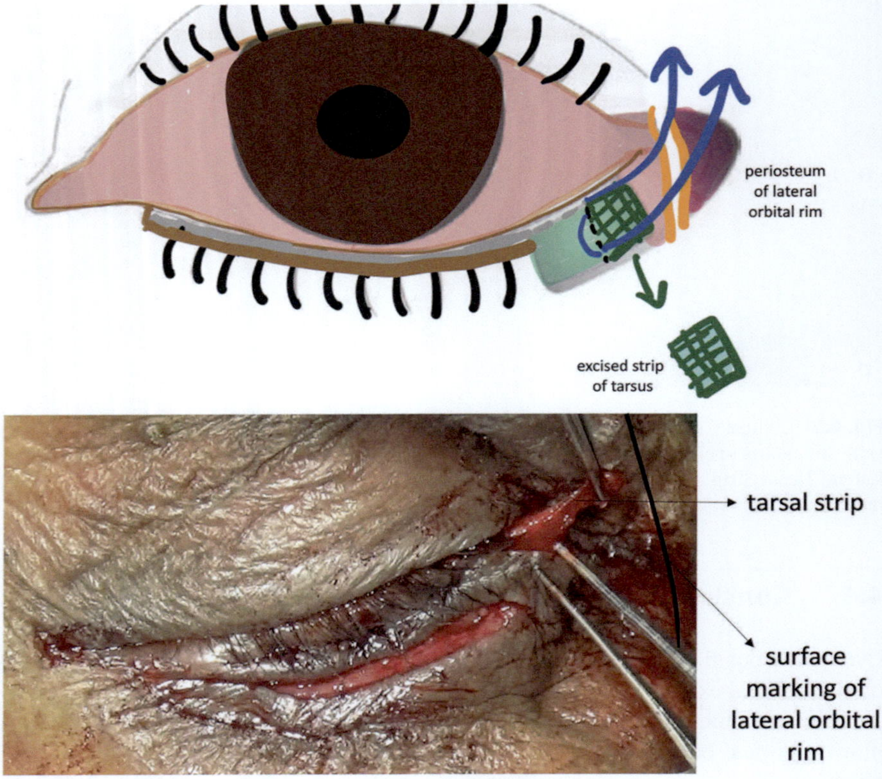

Fig. 4.10 Intraoperative steps for Lateral Tarsal Strip

inferior edge of the tarsal plate. The dissection is continued inferiorly to expose the conjunctiva. The orbital septum is opened and the orbital fat is retracted. The white line of disinserted retractors is identified. To confirm, the retractors are grasped in forceps and the patient is asked to look inferiorly, producing a tug. These are plicated and reattached to the inferior edge of the tarsus. Three to five such sutures are passed. The end point is slight eversion of eyelid without any stand-off. Additionally, crease forming sutures for lower eyelid crease and excess skin and orbicularis from inferior edge of incision may be excised if required.

Medial conjunctival spindle excision and retractor plication with inverting spiral suture for punctal inversion is required in medial ectropion without significant horizontal eyelid laxity, for relief of epiphora. Punctal snip for associated stenosis may be added. This is briefly described in Fig. 4.12. Under local anesthesia, the inferior canaliculus is identified and a Bowman's lacrimal probe is placed to protect it from iatrogenic injury. The eyelid is everted and a diamond (spindle) shaped piece of conjunctiva, and lower lid retractors is excised just inferior to the tarsus with the apex of the diamond in line with the punctum. An inverting spiral suture is then passed as follows. Both needles of a double-armed absorbable suture are passed

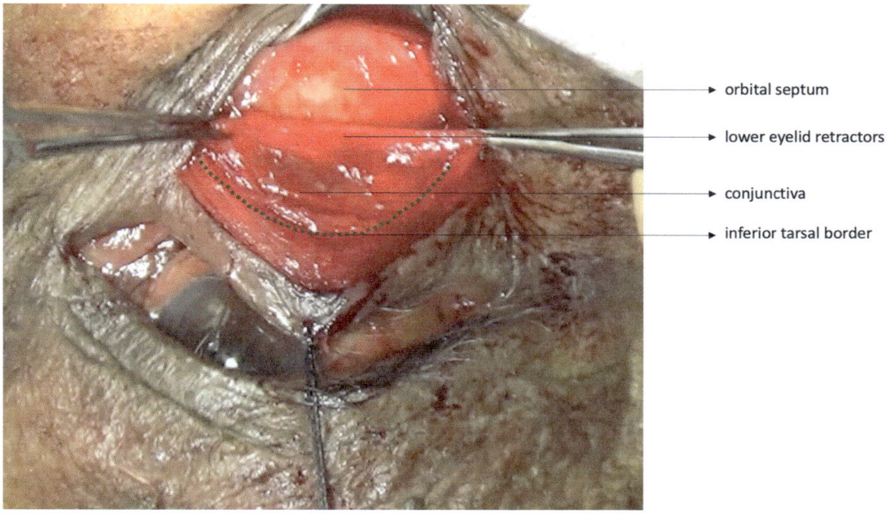

Fig. 4.11 Intraoperative steps for Jone's plication of inferior eyelid retractors

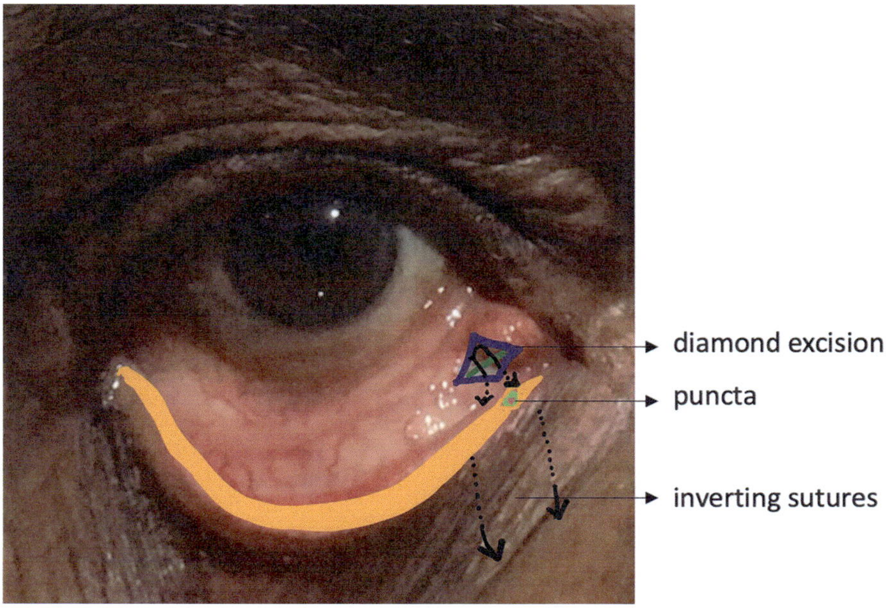

Fig. 4.12 Intraoperative steps for medial conjunctival spindle excision and retractor plication with inverting spiral suture for correcting the everted puncta

through the conjunctival opening engaging the lower lid retractors as follows. The needle bite is passed from inside the superior conjunctival edge then reversed and passed from inferior conjunctival edge to exit within the spindle while engaging the retractors (spiral suture). Both needles are then reversed and passed from within the spindle engaging the retractors, through the inferior border of tarsus and then exited through the eyelid skin and orbicularis close to the orbital rim to produce an inversion.

References

1. Kakizaki H, Malhotra R, Madge SN, Selva D. Lower eyelid anatomy: an update. Ann Plast Surg. 2009;63(3):344–51.
2. Kakizaki H, Zhao J, Nakano T, Asamoto K, Zako M, Iwaki M, Miyaishi O. The lower eyelid retractor consists of definite double layers. Ophthalmol. 2006;113:2346–50.
3. Bedran EG, Pereira MV, Bernardes TF. Ectropion. Semin Ophthalmol. 2010;25(3):59–65. https://doi.org/10.3109/08820538.2010.488570.
4. Adams AL. A case of double congenital ectropion. Med Fortnightly. 1896;9:137–8.
5. Imbert P. A theory of unified pathogenesis for tarsal ectropion and involutional entropion. J Fr Ophtalmol. 2020;43(7):611–7. https://doi.org/10.1016/j.jfo.2019.11.008.
6. Labib A, Patel BC, Milroy C. Lower eyelid laxity examination. In: StatPearls [Internet]. Treasure Island: StatPearls Publishing; 2022.
7. Moe KS, Linder T. The lateral transorbital canthopexy for correction and prevention of ectropion: report of a procedure, grading system, and outcome study. Arch Facial Plast Surg. 2000;2(1):9–15.
8. Anchlia S, Rao KS, Bonanthaya K, Anupama B, Nayak IV. Ophthalmic considerations in cleft lip and palate patients. J Maxillofac Oral Surg. 2011;10(1):14–9. https://doi.org/10.1007/s12663-010-0058-z.
9. Damasceno RW, Osaki MH, Dantas PE, Belfort R Jr. Involutional ectropion and entropion: clinicopathologic correlation between horizontal eyelid laxity and eyelid extracellular matrix. Ophthal Plast Reconstr Surg. 2011;27(5):321–6.
10. Kersten RC, Hammer BJ, Kulwin DR. The role of enophthalmos in involutional entropion. Ophthal Plast Reconstr Surg. 1997;13(3):195–8.
11. Kemp EG, Collin JR. Surgical management of upper lid entropion. Br J Ophthalmol. 1986;70:575–9.
12. Faria-e-Sousa SJ, Vieira MPG, Silva JV. Uncovering intermittent entropion. Clin Ophthalmol. 2013;7:385–38.
13. Kennedy AJ, Chowdhury H, Athwal S, Garg A, Baddeley P. Are you missing an entropion? The test of induced entropion 2. Ophthal Plast Reconstr Surg. 2015;31(6):437–9. https://doi.org/10.1097/iop.0000000000005.

Thyroid Eye Disease 5

Adit Gupta and Prerana Tahiliani

5.1 Case 1: Active Thyroid Eye Disease (TED) with No Optic Neuropathy

Classic TED presents with an active phase and a chronic inactive phase. The active phase ranges from 12 to 18 months followed by a more stable chronic phase in a typical disease course. In reality, not all patients go through the active phase or have a subclinical active phase. Active phase of the disease presents with dull pain, redness, eyelid retraction, proptosis, double vision, strabismus, and visual compromise in extreme cases. There are various grading systems to quantify the active phase of the disease, but lack of uniformity has always been a dilemma worldwide. Treatment has been mainly focused on symptomatic relief in the active phase, and research is ongoing to curtail this phase at the molecular level (Fig. 5.1) [1].

5.1.1 Case Summary

A 45-year-old male presented with swelling of both eyes with watering and photophobia. He also complained of weight loss and insomnia in the past few months. He was diagnosed with Graves' disease and started on medications. He developed eye symptoms simultaneously. On examination, he has eyelid edema with fluid malar bags, conjunctival chemosis. He also had mild proptosis with eyelid retraction and

A. Gupta (✉)
Mumbai Eye Plastic Surgery, Mumbai, India

P. Tahiliani
Mumbai Eye Plastic Surgery, Mumbai, India

Lotus Eye Hospital, Mumbai, India

A. Gupta, P. Tahiliani (eds.), *Oculoplastic and Orbit Casebook*, Current Practices in Ophthalmology, https://doi.org/10.1007/978-981-97-0593-1_5

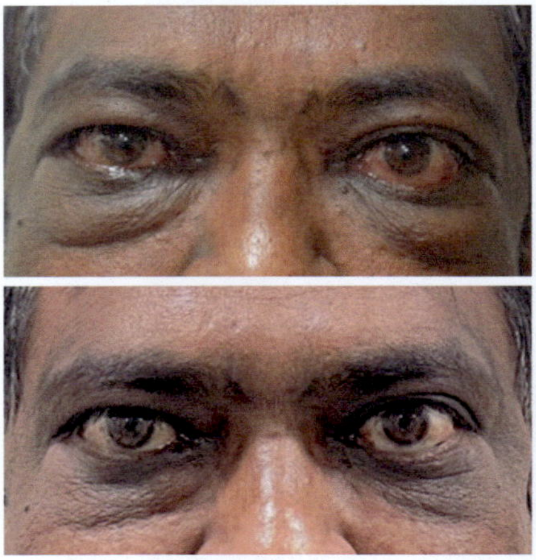

Fig. 5.1 Pre- and post-IV Methylprednisolone 6 doses. Note the improvement in edema, chemosis, and congestion of conjunctiva suggesting downstaging of the active disease

Table 5.1 Clinical activity score (CAS) by Mourits [2]. One point is given for each parameter assessed. Sum of parameters defines the clinical activity. Active ophthalmopathy if score > 3 in first exam or >4 in subsequent examination

	For initial CAS score items 1-7
1	Spontaneous orbital pain
2	Gaze evoked orbital pain
3	Eyelid swelling that is considered to be due to active GO
4	Eyelid erythema
5	Conjunctival redness considered due to active GO
6	Chemosis
7	Inflammation of caruncle or plica
	Follow-up after 1-3 months score items including 8-10
8	Increase of >2 mm proptosis
9	Decrease in uniocular ocular excursion in any one direction of >8 degrees
10	Decrease of acuity equivalent to 1 Snellen line

diplopia in primary gaze. His extraocular motility was restricted in up gaze. MRI revealed predominantly muscle disease with enlargement of extraocular muscles, but optic nerve compression was not noted. Clinically as well his vision was normal, and pupillary reflex was brisk with no relative afferent pupillary defect. He was diagnosed with active thyroid eye disease with a clinical activity score of 4 (in Table 5.1) and started on EUGOGO protocol (pulsed intravenous methylprednisolone-500 mg weekly 6 injections followed by 250 mg weekly 6 injections). He was kept under observation to note for any worsening of clinical picture.

At the end of 12 weeks, he had a significant improvement with resolution of eyelid edema and chemosis. His diplopia had resolved and the pain had subsided. He was kept under observation and is doing well at 1-year follow-up with good metabolic control.

5.1.2 Discussion

In case scenarios like this, where there is disease activity with classical signs of TED, steroids act as immunomodulators to shorten the disease course by controlling the disease activity. There are different protocols for steroid usage (EUGOGO protocol) [3] being the most followed internationally. Along with use of IV steroids, it is very important to stabilize the thyroid levels under the supervision of an endocrinologist. There is also a proven direct association between smoking and thyroid eye disease so smoking cessation plays an important role. Supportive eye care in the form of lubricant eye drops also provide relief from eye symptoms. Care has to be taken about the possible side effects of intravenous steroid use and vulnerable group patients (cardiac diseases, diabetics, osteoporosis, old age) should be monitored closely for any adverse effects.

5.2 Case 2: Active TED Resistant to Steroid Treatment

In certain cases, we see resistance to the efficacy of intravenous/oral steroids in the management of active disease. Some patients may show initial response followed by recurrence of symptoms and activity of the disease. These are usually case of resistant TED and are more commonly seen in male patients in the middle age group. Alternative treatments have to be thought of in such case scenarios (Fig. 5.2).

5.2.1 Case Summary

A 50-year-old male patient, smoker was treated for hyperthyroidism by an endocrinologist. He developed eye symptoms 6 months after the onset of eye disease in the form of proptosis and eyelid edema. He was prescribed intravenous steroids (cumulative dose 6 g) with minimal response. He presented with persistent swelling, restricted ocular motility, and caruncle edema to us. His vision and pupils were normal. Clinical activity score was 5. Considering his poor response to intravenous steroid, we decided to start him on oral immunosuppression. He was initiated on oral azathioprine under the supervision of a rheumatologist for a period of 1 year and was gradually tapered. He showed good response with resolution of his symptoms.

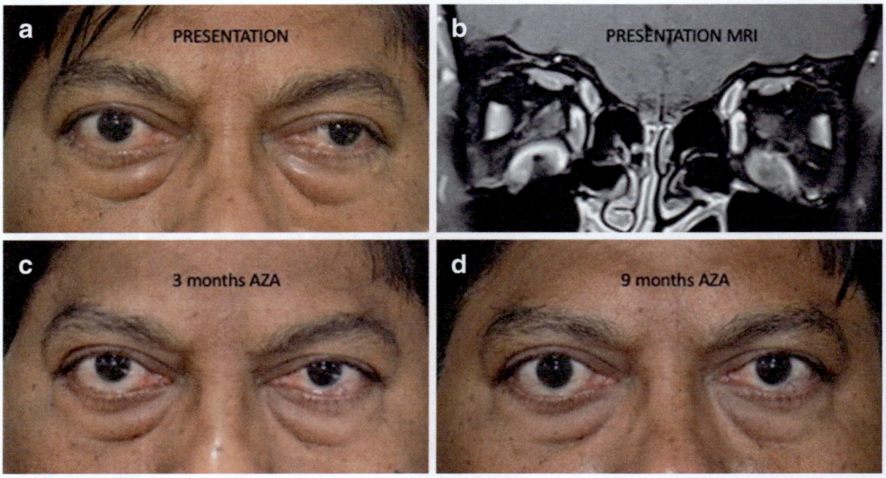

Fig. 5.2 Presentation picture showing eyelid edema, conjunctival chemosis with caruncle edema and strabismus; MRI image shows enlargement of muscles (inferior rectus); improvement can be noted 3 months after initiation of Azathioprine and at 9 months we note complete resolution of edema, chemosis, and strabismus. (**a**) At presentation; (**b**) MRI scan showing enlarged extraocular muscles with signs of activity (**c**) 3 months after oral Azathioprine showing partial resolution; (**d**) 9 months after oral immunotherapy showing almost complete resolution

5.2.2 Discussion

In case with poor or minimal response to steroids, immunosuppression has been tried as a rescue therapy with variable success. Various immunomodulators which have been used are azathioprine, mycophenolate, rituximab, tocilizumab, and adalimumab [4]. Recently, FDA has approved Teprotumumab, which targets IGF receptor for the treatment of thyroid eye disease in the United States. Studies have shown its efficacy in reducing the activity of disease and even proptosis in some cases. Long-term outcomes are yet to be known, but as of now this molecule shows maximum promise for the treatment of TED medically.

5.3 Case 3: TED with Sight-Threatening Optic Nerve Compression

Optic nerve compression is one of the rarest and severe complication of TED. Patient presents with rapidly deteriorating vision and loss of color perception. Of all the cases diagnosed with thyroid eye disease, less than 1% have signs of optic nerve compression. It is an ophthalmological emergency and medical followed by surgical decompression is mandated if a patient develops optic nerve compression secondary to TED (Fig. 5.3).

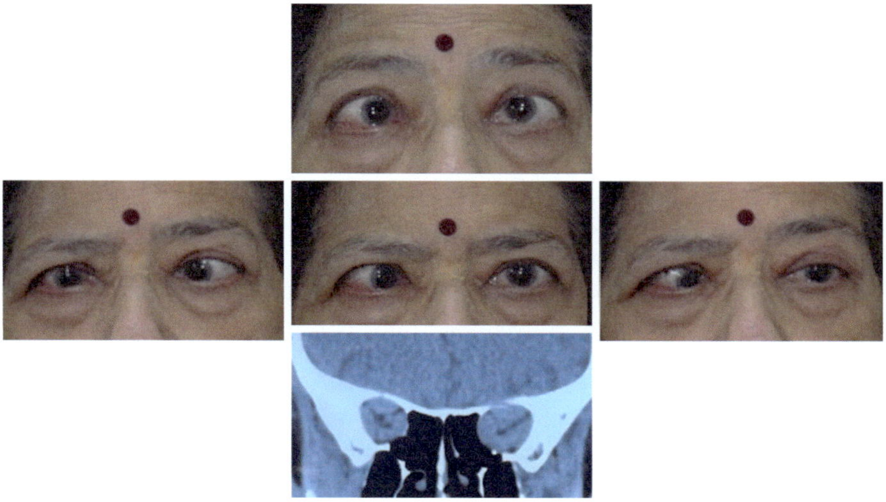

Fig. 5.3 A 60-year-old woman with central loss of vision and adduction. CT scan revealed compression of the optic nerve at the apex due to enlargement of extraocular muscles

5.3.1 Case Summary

A 63-year-old female was detected with hyperthyroidism and eye symptoms simultaneously. Her ocular symptoms were neglected due to the COVID pandemic, and she presented with decreased vision and severe strabismus 4 months after her symptoms began. On examination, she was amblyopic in one eye and the only seeing eye has counting fingers vision and afferent pupillary defect. She had lost color perception and had restrictive esotropia in the right eye. Imaging revealed enlargement of the extraocular muscles, especially the medial rectus with apical compression of the optic nerve.

She was started in intravenous steroids to reduce the pressure on the optic nerve. She had improvement in her vision after three steroid doses but deteriorated immediately after that. Endoscopic inferomedial orbital decompression was then performed to relieve the pressure on the orbital structures, and optic nerve was decompressed under visualization up to the orbital apex. Postoperatively she reported improvement in vision up to 6/60 and is under close observation.

5.3.2 Discussion

Optic nerve compression is an emergency situation and management have to be expedited in such cases. Dysthyroid optic neuropathy (DON) is associated with older age at presentation and has a male preponderance. There are different mechanisms proposed for the neuropathy which include disturbance of axoplasmic flow due to compression, stretching of the optic nerve and inflammation. The most common presenting symptom is blurring of central vision and color desaturation. A relative afferent pupillary defect is noted if it is asymmetric. Proptosis is not a characteristic feature in patients developing DON. Visual field defects are noted in some patients. Medical decompression in the form of immediate intravenous steroids should be initiated till the time the patient can be prepared for surgery. Surgery is a more definitive way to relieve the compression on the optic nerve. Medial and inferior wall decompression are traditionally performed in such cases. Surgery can be performed via the trans-caruncular approach to open up the lamina papyracea. The advantage of this approach is quicker surgical time and lesser instrumentation. Endoscopic medial wall decompression although more complicated has the advantage of direct visualization of structures and possibility of reaching the orbital apex as well. Necessary training in endoscopic procedures and a more expensive setup is needed to perform endoscopic decompression. If detected and treated in time, these patients have a very good visual prognosis (Table 5.2).

Table 5.2 Management of DON

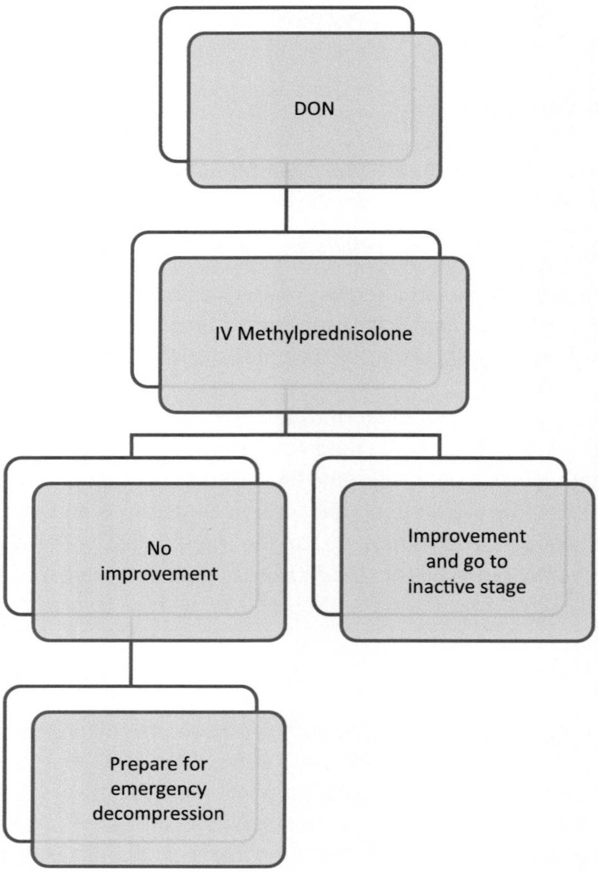

5.3.3 Caution

Radioactive iodine (RAI) is a known treatment for hyperthyroidism. In some patients, the ocular symptoms may worsen after radiation-RAI, and vision can worsen caused by optic nerve compromise. It is hypothesized that RAI releases thyroid antigens that are then directed toward the orbit. As a general recommendation, the patients who are scheduled to receive RAI, are placed on pre-RAI steroids. This is important in patients that have pre-existing eye disease with enlarged muscles (medial rectus) close to the optic nerve.

5.4 Case 4: Burnt Out TED

It is common to find a patient with TED presenting directly with burnt out disease. The patient does not present with characteristic signs of active phase but will present with eyelid retraction or with proptosis and a white eye. These patients are usually the ones who have been overprescribed on steroids by the general ophthalmologists mistaking it with active disease. Identifying this subgroup of patients is very important to avoid unnecessary medication. These are the patients who mainly need functional and cosmetic rehabilitation.

5.4.1 Case Summary

A 30-year-old female had unilateral proptosis for some years. She was diagnosed with hypothyroidism and was on treatment. Multiple courses of oral steroids were prescribed in hope of reducing the proptosis. The other eye was normal. The affected eye had normal vision and demonstrated severe proptosis with eyelid retraction. Clinical activity score was 0. There were no signs of inflammation. CT scan revealed fat predominant disease with minimal involvement of muscles. She was observed over a 3-month period for stability of disease. Previous photos were assessed to see the progression over years. She was bothered by the cosmetic appearance of her eyes due to the stark asymmetry. Balanced orbital decompression was performed along with fat decompression and 6 mm reduction of proptosis was achieved as seen in Fig. 5.4. Eyelid lengthening procedure was performed for the upper eyelid by recessing the levator muscle to achieve optimal eyelid symmetry after 6 weeks.

5.4.2 Discussion

Asymmetric proptosis and eyelid retraction are the two most disfiguring sequelae of chronic TED. Apart from functional indications they can be cosmetically disfiguring and need corrective surgery. Surgical approaches are now minimally invasive with less morbidity and complications. Stepwise approach is preferred to correct and the order followed is [5]:

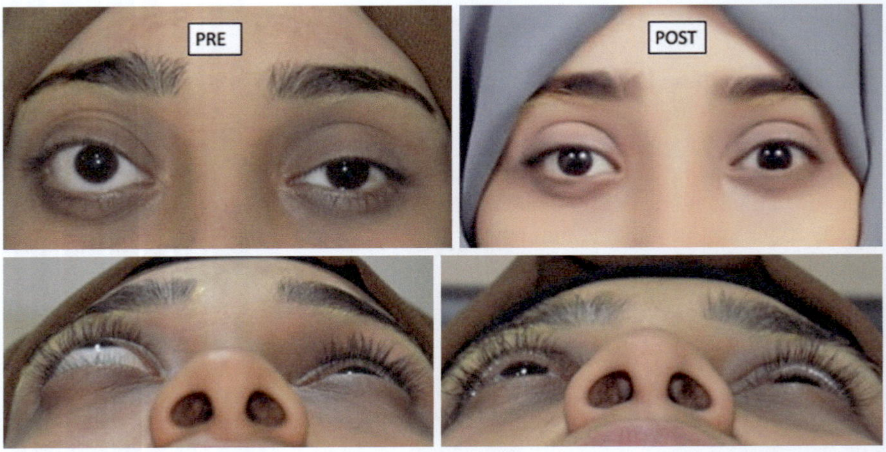

Fig. 5.4 A 30-year-old hypothyroid girl had asymmetric proptosis with eyelid retraction. She had no signs of active eye disease. She underwent orbital decompression surgery to reposition the eyeball followed by an eyelid recession surgery to lower the eyelid. Final outcome is seen at 3 months after the procedures

1. Orbital decompression to reduce proptosis.
2. Strabismus correction if any.
3. Eyelid surgery to correct retraction.
4. Cosmetic surgery/blepharoplasty for sculpting the periocular tissues.

New onset diplopia is the commonest complication following orbital decompression and the incidence has reduced over the years by using modern techniques. Surgery is not a definitive treatment, but till we invent a biologic agent which targets the disease process at the molecular level it forms the mainstay for rehabilitating these patients.

5.4.3 Conclusion

Thyroid eye disease needs multifactorial management with close coordination between an ophthalmologist, endocrinologist, and rheumatologist. It is very important to control the thyroid hormone levels to effectively manage the eye disease. Immunomodulators offer promise to control this disease at the molecular level and obviate the need for surgery. Teprotumumab is the latest drug which offers promise to control this disease than previously tried medicines but needs to stand the test of time and affordability is another roadblock. Till we have a definitive therapy, surgical correction of sequelae is the only option for this disease.

Conflict of Interest The authors have no financial interests and the photos have been displayed with proper patient consent and permission.

References

1. Kahaly GJ. Immunotherapies for thyroid eye disease. Curr Opin Endocrinol Diabetes Obes. 2019;26(5):250–5.
2. Mourits MP, Prummel MF, Wiersinga WM, Koornneef L. Clinical activity score as a guide in the management of patients with Graves' ophthalmopathy. Clin Endocrinol. 1997;47(1):9–14.
3. Bartalena L, Kahaly GJ, Baldeschi L, Dayan CM, Eckstein A, Marcocci C, Marinò M, Vaidya B, Wiersinga WM, EUGOGO. The 2021 European Group on Graves' orbitopathy (EUGOGO) clinical practice guidelines for the medical management of Graves' orbitopathy. Eur J Endocrinol. 2021;185(4):G43–67.
4. Douglas RS, Gupta S. The pathophysiology of thyroid eye disease: implications for immunotherapy. Curr Opin Ophthalmol. 2011;22(5):385–90.
5. Naik MN, Nair AG, Gupta A, Kamal S. Minimally invasive surgery for thyroid eye disease. Indian J Ophthalmol. 2015;63(11):847–5.

Acute Dacryocystitis and Sequelae

6

Nandini Bothra and Ayushi Agarwal

6.1 Introduction

Acute dacryocystitis is defined as "a medical urgency which is clinically characterized by rapid onset of pain, erythema and swelling, classically below the medial canthal tendon with or without pre-existing epiphora, mainly resulting from the acute infection of the lacrimal sac and perisac tissues" [1]. The prevalence of acute dacryocystitis is about 2.4% of all lacrimal disorders. It is usually seen in the third to fifth decades of life and has a female preponderance.

6.2 Microbiology

Microbiological profile is mainly [2]:

1. Gram-positive cocci—56%—Commonest isolates are *Staphylococcus aureus*, *Streptococcus pneumoniae*, and *Streptococcus pyogenes*.
2. Gram-negative bacilli—30%—Common isolates are *Hemophilus influenzae*, *Escherichia coli*, and *Pseudomonas aeruginosa*.
3. Gram-positive bacilli—3%.
4. Sterile cultures have been noted in approximately 11% of cases.

N. Bothra (✉) · A. Agarwal
Govindram Seksaria Institute of Dacryology, Ophthalmic Plastic Surgery Services, LV Prasad Eye Institute, Hyderabad, India

A. Gupta, P. Tahiliani (eds.), *Oculoplastic and Orbit Casebook*, Current Practices in Ophthalmology, https://doi.org/10.1007/978-981-97-0593-1_6

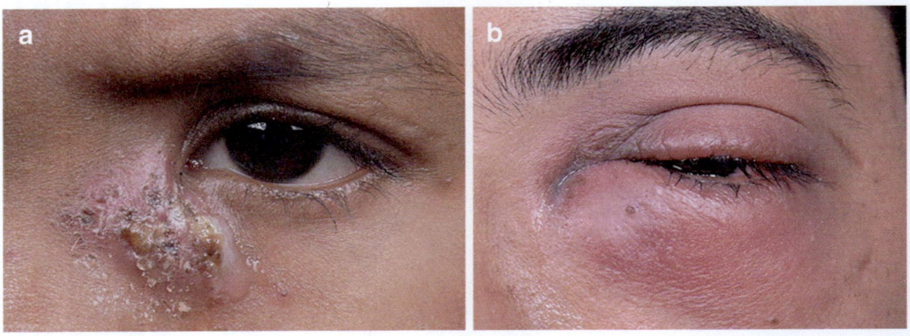

Fig. 6.1 Clinical photograph of a 10-year-old child with left-sided acute dacryocystitis (Panel A). Clinical photograph showing left-sided acute dacryocystitis which progressed to pre-septal cellulitis (Panel B)

6.3 Clinical Presentation: (Fig. 6.1)

Symptoms:

1. Pain.
2. Swelling in the lacrimal area, sometimes involving the entire lower eyelid usually below the medial canthal tendon.
3. Redness.
4. Watering.
5. Discharge—mucoid to mucopurulent.

Signs:

1. Tender swelling in the lacrimal sac area.
2. Warm to touch.
3. High tear meniscus height.
4. Discharge.
5. Regurgitation of purulent material from the puncta.
6. Other signs like the presence of an abscess and discharging fistula, swelling of the lower and upper eyelid, conjunctival congestion, proptosis, external ophthalmoplegia, and diminution or loss of vision can be seen if the inflammation progresses to involve the periorbital and periocular tissues.

6.4 Complications/Progression

Acute dacryocystitis can progress to involve the periocular and periorbital tissues and lead to:

1. Pre-septal cellulitis.
2. Lacrimal abscess.

3. Lacrimal fistula.
4. Orbital cellulitis.
5. Orbital abscess.
6. Necrotizing fasciitis.
7. Superior ophthalmic vein thrombosis.
8. Central/branched retina artery occlusion.
9. Cavernous sinus thrombosis.
10. Meningitis.

Lacrimal abscess, fistula, and pre-septal cellulitis are the most common complications of acute dacryocystitis.

6.5 Management

The ultimate goal of treatment is to relieve the nasolacrimal duct obstruction which can be achieved only by surgical techniques.

1. Conservative management.

   Conservative management is temporary and is aimed to relieve the pain and buy time till surgical intervention can be planned. It consists of warm compresses, systemic antibiotics based on common regional isolates and sensitivity profiles, and anti-inflammatory drugs. Resolution occurs in about 7–10 days.

   Non-resolving acute dacryocystitis can be due to:
   (a) Lacrimal abscess/fistula formation.
   (b) Antibiotic resistance.
   (c) Virulent organism.
2. Surgical management [3, 4].

   This is the mainstay of treatment. After control of acute infection, dacryocystorhinostomy can be planned. External or endoscopic approach would depend on the surgeon and either technique has shown similar success rates (>90%).

   The advantages of endoscopic approach in acute infections:
   (a) Can be done in the acute stage.
   (b) Avoidance of skin incision, thus, less bleeding and no scar formation.
   (c) Faster relief of pain as can be done in the acute stage.
   (d) Postoperative comfort and early rehabilitation.

6.6 Case 1

A 33-year-old farmer presented to the dacryology clinic with complaints of pain, redness, and swelling in the lacrimal sac area of the right eye of 3-day duration (Fig. 6.2, Panel A). The swelling showed regurgitation of mucopurulent discharge from the puncta on pressure. The patient was diagnosed to have bilateral cicatrizing conjunctivitis about a year ago; hence, the ocular surface was dry and there was no history of epiphora. Occurrence of a single episode of acute dacryocystitis in the

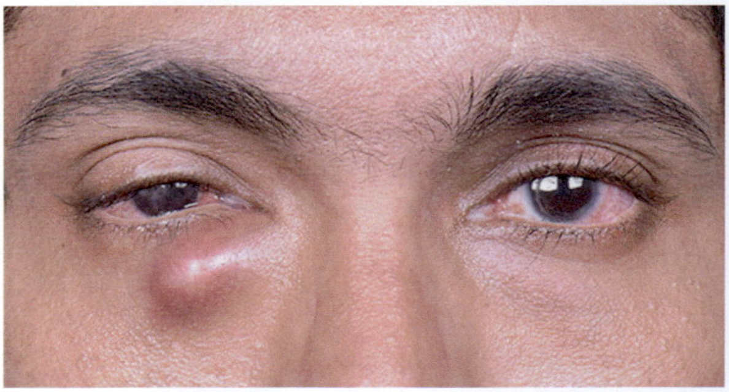

Fig. 6.2 Clinical photograph of Case 1 showing a right-sided tender swelling which is anterior, inferior, and lateral to the presumed sac area, raising a suspicion of diverticulitis with associated acute dacryocystitis

past was elicited. On examination, there was a tender swelling in the lacrimal sac area, below the medial canthal tendon. However, the swelling was much more lateral, inferior, and anterior in position, which increased in size on irrigation, pointing towards a possibility of acute dacryocystitis with diverticulitis (Fig. 6.2). Schirmer's test confirmed bilateral severe dry eye disease (DED).

Considering severe DED secondary to cicatrizing conjunctivitis warranting hourly lubricant instillation, dacryocystectomy (DCT) with diverticulectomy was opted and performed. Histopathology of the diverticula tissue showed a dilated lumen lined by stratified columnar epithelium with goblet cells. The stroma showed chronic inflammatory cells. The patient's ocular surface is stable with no bothersome epiphora at 1-year follow-up.

6.6.1 Discussion [5–7]

Lacrimal diverticula are outpouchings from the canaliculi or the lacrimal sac, occurring secondary to a weakness in the wall due to either repeated inflammations, trauma, or sometimes congenital origin. Diverticula most commonly arises from the lacrimal sac followed by canaliculi. Lateral diverticula are the most preferred location as the sac is only covered by periorbital laterally, thus offering the least resistance to the sac in that direction. The opening of the diverticulum within the lacrimal drainage apparatus is small and usually acts as a one-way valve, leading to stagnation of secretions in the diverticula cavity. This collection of secretions in the cavity makes it more prone to develop an acute infection. Dacryoliths (mucopeptide concretions) may also form in the diverticula cavity.

Diagnosis of lacrimal sac diverticulum is generally with a dacryocystogram (DCG) where filling of the cavity can be noted. It may or may not be associated with a nasolacrimal duct obstruction. Treatment is primarily surgical, depending upon the presence or absence of nasolacrimal duct obstruction. Patent lacrimal system with diverticula can be managed with a simple diverticulectomy, taking due precautions to avoid damage to the lacrimal drainage system. Association of diverticula with nasolacrimal duct obstruction can be managed with a dacryocystorhinostomy (external or endoscopic) with complete diverticulectomy or marsupialization of the cavity with enlargement of the cavity opening into the lacrimal sac [8].

6.7 Case 2

A 33-year-old male presented to the clinic with painful swelling along the upper and lower eyelid of the left eye, associated with sudden loss of vision for 3 days. A history of watering and discharge for 1 month prior to the development of swelling was elicited. The patient had received a course of oral acetazolamide from elsewhere. Right eye examination was unremarkable. The left eye vision was nil perception of light (NPL). Ocular motility was limited in all gazes with associated ptosis and chemosis. (Fig. 6.3, Panel A). Fundoscopy revealed central retinal artery occlusion (CRAO), which was eventually attributed to orbital cellulitis. Computed Tomography (CT) scan of the orbits showed heterogenous lesion involving the lacrimal sac region, pre-septal area, and medial orbit extending up to mid-orbit. Subperiosteal abscess formation was seen in the medial orbit (Fig. 6.3, Panel B). A provisional diagnosis of orbital cellulitis with subperiosteal abscess formation and central retinal artery occlusion, secondary to acute dacryocystitis was established.

Patient was admitted for medical management and was started on intravenous antibiotics and analgesics and was scheduled for abscess drainage the next day. The abscess was drained and the aspirate was sent for microbiological analysis, which revealed significant growth of *Staphylococcus aureus* and *Pseudomonas aeruginosa*, resistant to all fluoroquinolones and azithromycin. The patient was started on intravenous antibiotics based on antibiotic sensitivity pattern along with intravenous steroids to help resolution of inflammation. The swelling reduced over the next 3 days with restoration of motility and resolution of chemosis. However, the vision could not be recovered owing to CRAO (Fig. 6.3, Panel C). Following resolution of orbital cellulitis, irrigation findings confirmed the presence of nasolacrimal obstruction following which a dacryocystorhinostomy was performed.

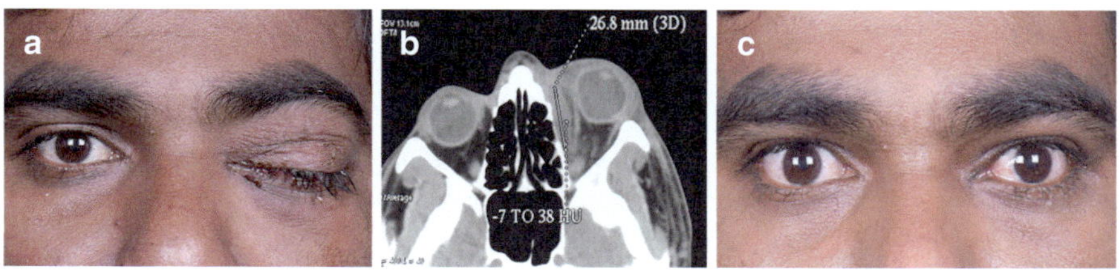

Fig. 6.3 Clinical photograph of Case 2 at presentation, revealing features of orbital cellulitis (Panel A). CT scan of the orbit, axial view, showing heterogenous lesion involving the lacrimal sac with orbital extension upto the mid-orbit. Subperiosteal abscess formation is noted in the medial orbit (Panel B). Clinical photograph of Case 2 showing complete resolution of orbital cellulitis and acute dacryocystitis following intravenous antibiotics, steroids and drainage of the abscess (Panel C)

6.7.1 Discussion [9–14]

As mentioned above, acute dacryocystitis can often lead to pre-septal cellulitis and formation of lacrimal abscess and fistula. However, strong anatomical barriers like the deep heads of pre-septal and pretarsal orbicularis, lacrimal fascia, insertions of orbital septum and medial canthal ligament at the lacrimal crest prevent the spread of infection to the orbit. Long-standing infection or repeated attacks of acute inflammation may weaken this barrier and aid in the spread of infection to and beyond the orbit. Other modes of spread include via the ethmoid sinus and lamina papyracea or hematogenous spread in selected cases. Increase in the intraorbital pressure secondary to inflammation can lead to retinal vein and artery occlusions.

Once the infection spreads to the orbit, the primary aim is to control the infection and then manage the nasolacrimal duct obstruction secondarily. Intravenous medications are the preferred route of drug delivery and intravenous steroids hasten the resolution of inflammation. Microbiology and sensitivity profile helps in tailoring the medications to achieve swift response.

References

1. Ali MJ, Joshi DS, Naik MN, et al. Clinical profile and management outcome of acute dacryocystitis: two decades of experience in a tertiary eye care center. Semin Ophthalmol. 2015;30:118–23.
2. Ali MJ, Motukupally SR, Joshi SD, et al. The microbiological profile of lacrimal abscess: two decades of experience from a tertiary eye care center. J Ophthalmic Inflamm Infect. 2013;3:57–61.
3. Kamal S, Ali MJ, Pujari A, et al. Primary powered endoscopic dacryocystorhinostomy in the setting of acute dacryocystitis and lacrimal abscess. Ophthal Plast Reconstr Surg. 2015;31:293–5.
4. Jain S, Ganguly A, Singh S, et al. Primary non-endoscopic endonasal versus delayed external dacryocystorhinostomy in acute dacryocystitis. Ophthal Plast Reconstr Surg. 2016;33:285–8.
5. Sinnreich Z. Lacrimal diverticula. Orbit. 1998;17:195–200.
6. Ali MJ, Naik MN. Congenital lacrimal sac diverticulum. Saudi J Ophthalmol. 2017;31:199–200.
7. Cnaan RB, Abumanhal M, Wengier A, Feldman I, Leibovitch I, Abergel A. Lacrimal sac diverticulum: clinical presentation and endoscopic management. Eur Arch Otorhinolaryngol. 2022;279:199–203.
8. Ali MJ. Endoscopic approach to management of a lacrimal sac diverticula. Ophthalmic Plast Reconstr Surg. 2016;32:e49.
9. Bothra N, Agarwal K, Ali MJ. Panophthalmitis and visual loss as a complication of acute dacryocystitis. Ophthalmic Plast Reconstr Surg. 2020;36:e156–8.
10. Maheshwari R, Maheshwari S, Shah T. Acute dacryocystitis causing orbital cellulitis and abscess. Orbit. 2009;28:196–9.
11. Kikkawa DO, Heinz GW, Martin RT, Nunery WN, Eiseman AS. Orbital cellulitis and abscess secondary to dacryocystitis. Arch Ophthalmol. 2002;120(8):1096–9.
12. Pfeiffer ML, Hacopian A, Merritt H, Phillips ME, Richani K. Complete vision loss following orbital cellulitis secondary to acute dacryocystitis. Case Rep Ophthalmol Med. 2016;2016:9630698.
13. Ahrens-Palumbo MJ, Ballen PH. Primary dacryocystitis causing orbital cellulitis. Ann Ophthalmol. 1982;14:600–1.
14. Bothra N, Tyagi M, Ali MJ. Central retinal artery occlusion as a complication of acute dacryocystitis. Int Ophthalmol Clin. 2023;63(3):187–.93. https://doi.org/10.1097/IIO.0000000000000472.

Secondary Acquired Nasolacrimal Duct Obstruction

7

Nandini Bothra and Ayushi Agarwal

7.1 Introduction

Bartley in 1992 coined the term secondary acquired lacrimal duct obstruction (SALDO) to describe nasolacrimal obstructions for which specific cause is known. He classified it into five categories: Traumatic, Infectious, Inflammatory, Mechanical, and Neoplastic [1]. The management of SALDO depends upon recognising and addressing the underlying causative entity.

7.2 Case 1

A 27-year-old male presented to the clinic with painful swelling in the right lower lid for the past 1 week. A history of constant watering and discharge of 3-year duration in the right eye following a road-traffic accident (RTA) was elicited. Immediately following trauma, the patient underwent maxillofacial repair, which was followed 6 months later by nasal implant placement and revision of the repaired facial fracture, elsewhere. Subsequently, the nasal implant got infected and hence, was removed. At presentation, the patient was already on oral antibiotics (Tablet amoxicillin + clavulanic acid 625 mg twice a day) for 4 days which had led to significant relief in pain and redness. On examination, a right-sided non-tender swelling in the medial canthal area and medial lower eyelid was noted with an associated acquired fistula (Fig. 7.1, Panel A). Extraocular movements, pupillary reflex, and fundoscopy were within normal limits. Depressed nasal bridge and telecanthus were present. A working diagnosis of resolving acute dacryocystitis secondary to traumatic SALDO was established. A Computed Tomography (CT) scan of the Orbit and Paranasal Sinuses

N. Bothra (✉) · A. Agarwal
Govindram Seksaria Institute of Dacryology, Ophthalmic Plastic Surgery Services, LV Prasad Eye Institute, Hyderabad, India

A. Gupta, P. Tahiliani (eds.), *Oculoplastic and Orbit Casebook*, Current Practices in Ophthalmology, https://doi.org/10.1007/978-981-97-0593-1_7

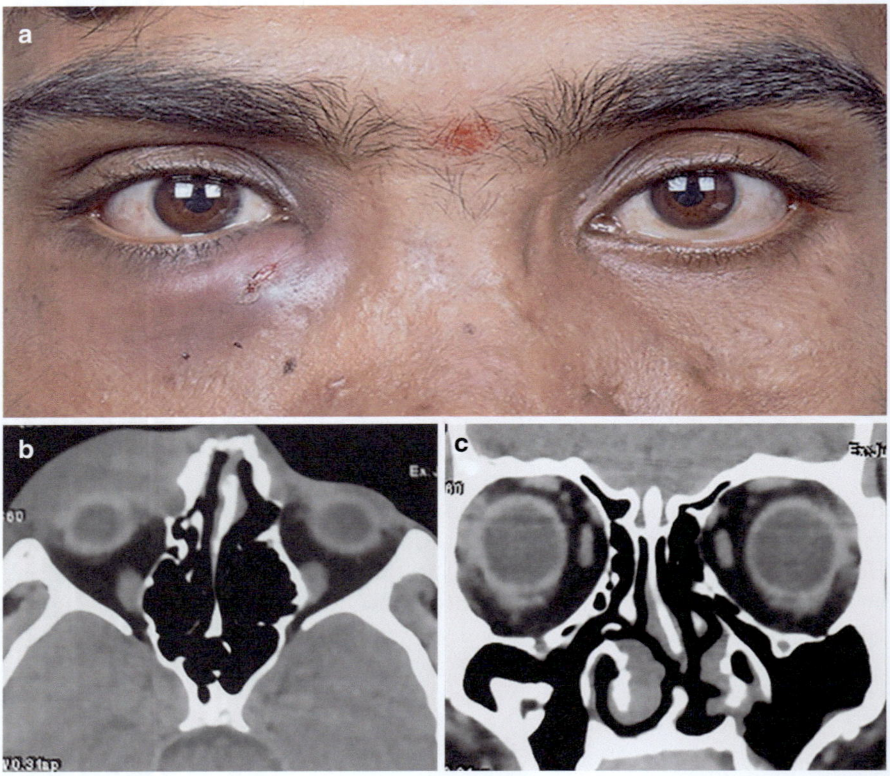

Fig. 7.1 Clinical photograph of Case 1, showing right medial canthal swelling with acquired lacrimal fistula and associated skin changes (Panel **a**). CT Scan, axial view, soft tissue window showing isodense lesion in the right lacrimal fossa region extending to the pre-septal space (Panel **b**). Coronal view, bone window, revealing anterior nasal septal defect, hypertrophied right inferior turbinate with DNS toward the left side (Panel **c**)

revealed features of right-sided lacrimal sac swelling extending along the preseptal space. Fractures of the right lacrimal sac fossa and bony nasolacrimal duct (NLD) were noted. An anterior nasal septal defect with hypertrophied ipsilateral inferior turbinate and deviated nasal septum towards the left side were revealed. Cribriform plate appeared intact with no visualization of maxillofacial implants or associated orbital wall fractures (Fig. 7.1, Panel B and C). A pre-operative nasal endoscopy revealed multiple synechiae at the level of anterior nares with grossly altered nasal anatomy on the right side, rendering the endoscopic maneuvering challenging.

Considering the extensively distorted nasal architecture with septal defect, and history of prior nasal infection, a decision to perform external dacryocystorhinostomy (DCR) with mitomycin-C (MMC) and silicone tube intubation was made. The surgery was uneventful with complete subjective and anatomical resolution at 1-month follow-up.

7.3 Case 2

A 31-year-old male presented to the clinic with watering and discharge from the right eye following RTA of 3-year duration. There was history of prior maxillofacial, frontal bone, and dural tear repair. On examination, facial asymmetry along with bilateral telecanthus was noted with mucopurulent regurgitation on pressure over lacrimal sac (ROPLAS positive) on the right side (Fig. 7.2, Panel A). The lacrimal irrigation on the left side was freely patent. No evidence of enophthalmos or hypoglobus was seen. A three-dimensional CT- Dacryocystography (3D CT-DCG) revealed a dilated sac fairly in position, with obstruction at the sac-duct junction. Right-sided naso-orbito-ethmoid (NOE) fracture, multiple plates and screws on both sides for the underlying zygomatic and maxillary fractures, and a low-lying fractured cribriform plate were noted (Fig. 7.2, Panel B–D). A pre-operative nasal endoscopy revealed normal nasal anatomy. A diagnosis of right-sided traumatic SALDO was established and an endoscopic DCR with silicone tube intubation was performed. Intra-operatively, caution was exercised due to extensive fractures of the facial bones and cribriform plate. Instead of using bone rongeur's, bone drilling was preferred to reduce the torsion as well as the pull over the nasal bones and hence,

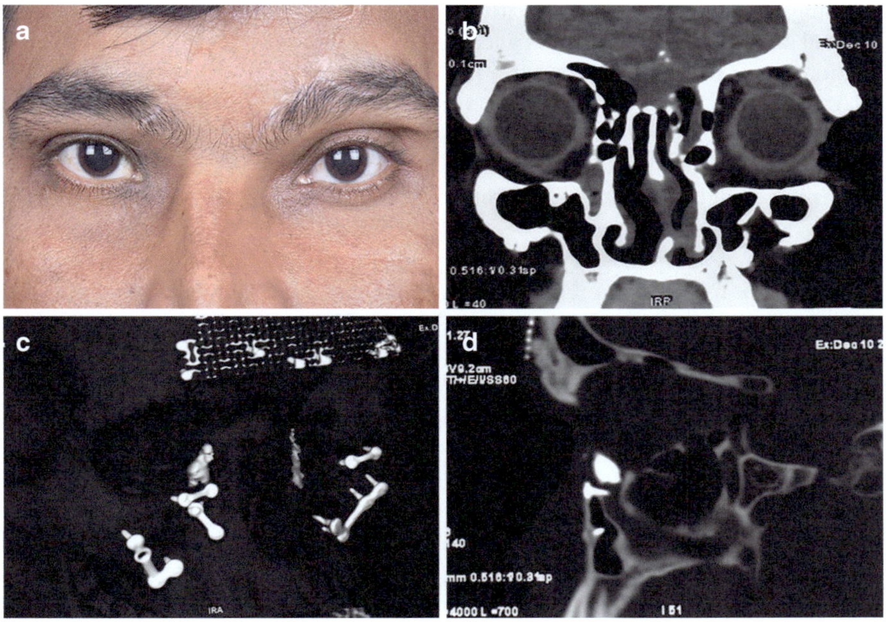

Fig. 7.2 Clinical photograph of Case 2 showing facial asymmetry and bilateral telecanthus following trauma (Panel A). CT scan, coronal view, soft tissue window, showing multiple nasal fractures (Panel B). 3D CT-DCG shows right dilated sac in normal position with abrupt cessation of dye uptake at sac-duct junction, along with multiple plates and screws in close vicinity of the sac (Panel C), as also highlighted in the parasagittal section (Panel D)

avoid cerebrospinal fluid (CSF) leak and dural damage. At 1-month follow-up, the stent was extubated and the anatomical patency along with symptomatic resolution was achieved.

7.3.1 Discussion

Traumatic SALDO is a common, yet a challenging entity. Epiphora due to traumatic SALDO can occur shortly or even years after trauma, due to the intense inflammation and cicatrizing reaction. The most significant cause is an NOE fracture as they can have an associated lacrimal fossa fracture or NLD dehiscence. However, factors like direct lacrimal sac laceration, multiple facial fractures, and prior iatrogenic trauma may also be causative [2].

Endoscopic DCR is the author's preferred choice for managing primary acquired nasolacrimal duct obstruction with comparable success rates as the external approach, scarless outcomes, and early post-operative rehabilitation. However, in cases of traumatic SALDO, features such as distorted nasal architecture including disturbed relationship of middle turbinate (MT) with lacrimal sac or bulla ethmoidalis, low-lying or damaged cribriform plate, concomitant skull base fractures, breach in the periorbita, and nasal septum alterations, should be considered prior to planning an endoscopic approach [3]. In these challenging situations, navigation-assisted dacryolocalization helps in accurately determining the anatomic and spatial relationship of the relevant structures [4].

Alternatively, an external approach may be preferred in situations of altered nasal anatomy and compromised endoscopic view. Other relative indications include the presence of lacrimal diverticula, simultaneous orbital intervention, or concurrent skull base injury with higher risk of intra-operative CSF leak.

An endoscopic DCR may be preferred over an external DCR in the presence of multiple screws and plates in the vicinity of the lacrimal sac secondary to previous facial fracture repair, scarring of the tissues, and extensive bony callous formation in the tear trough region.

In conclusion, a comprehensive history and examination, relevant lacrimal imaging, and a pre-operative endoscopic nasal evaluation is vital in all cases of traumatic SALDO to decide the optimal surgical procedure, anticipate possible intra-operative complications, and determine the prognosis.

7.4 Case 3

A 76-year-old female presented with painless swelling in the left medial canthal area of 3 months duration with associated epiphora. A prior functional endoscopic sinus surgery was performed an year ago elsewhere for skull base lesion of presumed fungal etiology. Examination revealed a firm palpable mass below the medial canthal ligament, along with superolateral displacement of the left globe (Fig. 7.3, Panel A). ROPLAS was negative. CT scan orbit and paranasal sinus revealed an isodense, well-defined lesion with epicenter in the lacrimal fossa, extending into the ipsilateral inferomedial orbit, ethmoid sinus, as well as frontal sinus with no bony erosion (Fig. 7.3, Panel B). A provisional diagnosis of lacrimal sac granuloma was made, with lacrimal sac malignancy kept as another differential diagnosis. The lesion was debulked and sent for histopathological evaluation, which revealed filamentous, acute-angled, branching fungal hyphae with positive Gomori methenamine silver staining, definitive of an aspergilloma. Post-operatively, the patient was started on anti-fungal medications (Tablet Voriconazole 200 mg twice/day) for 1 month, which resulted in complete clinical resolution of the lesion (Fig. 7.3, Panel C). This was followed by maintenance dose of Tab Itraconazole 100 mg twice/day for 3 months. No recurrence was noted at 4-month follow-up.

7.4.1 Discussion

The above is a case of an infectious SALDO, resulting due to a lacrimal sac granuloma of fungal etiology.

Lacrimal sac fungal granuloma is a rare entity, which usually presents as a unilateral medial canthal swelling, with or without features of nasolacrimal duct obstruction. The closest differential diagnosis in the above case was a lacrimal sac malignancy. However, the absence of hemolacria, history of prior skull base lesions of fungal etiology, absence of mass extension beyond medial canthal tendon, and absent lymphadenopathy were the few clinical pointers against a lacrimal sac malignancy [5]. Intra-operatively during debulking, the lesion appeared to arise from the sac itself with orbital and sinus extension.

Considering the endemicity of tuberculosis (TB) in the Indian subcontinent, lacrimal sac granuloma secondary to TB should be kept as another differential diagnosis. To distinguish, histopathological evaluation (HPE) remains the gold standard for diagnosis. Fungal aspergillus granuloma mandates debulking or excision of the lesion with prompt initiation of anti-fungal therapy, namely oral voriconazole and itraconazole. Long-term follow-up is recommended as recurrence is a possibility [6].

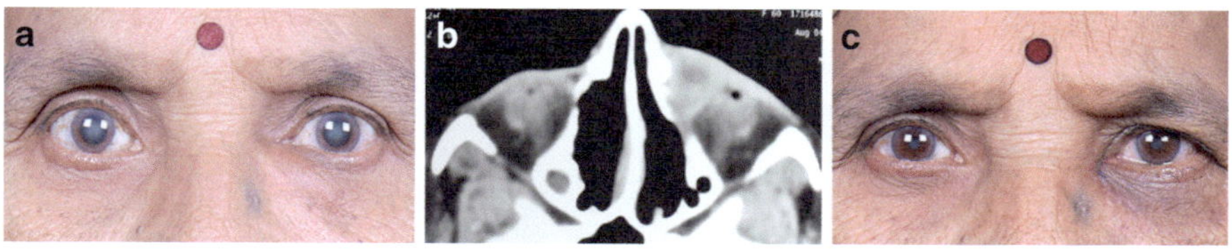

Fig. 7.3 Clinical photograph of Case 3, showing left painless, medial canthal swelling with superolateral displacement of the left globe (Panel A). CT Scan, axial view, showing isodense lesion in the left lacrimal fossa without bony erosion and orbital and sinus extension (Panel B). Clinical resolution of the lesion following excision biopsy and initiation of oral anti-fungal therapy at post-operative 1-week period (Panel C)

References

1. Bartley GB. Acquired lacrimal drainage obstruction: an etiologic classification system, case reports, and a review of the literature. Part 1. Ophthalmic. Plast Reconstr Surg. 1992;8(4):237–42.
2. Mukherjee B, Dhobekar M. Traumatic nasolacrimal duct obstruction: clinical profile, management, and outcome. Eur J Ophthalmol. 2013;23(5):615–22.
3. Ali MJ, Naik MN. Image-guided dacryolocalization (IGDL) in traumatic secondary acquired lacrimal drainage obstructions (SALDO). Ophthalmic Plast Reconstr Surg. 2015;31(5):406–9.
4. Ali MJ. Disorders of the upper lacrimal system. In: Ali MJ, editor. Principles and practice of lacrimal surgery. 2nd ed. Singapore: Springer; 2018. p. 133–40.
5. Pao KY, Yakopson V, Flanagan JC, Eagle RC Jr. Allergic fungal sinusitis involving the lacrimal sac: a case report and review. Orbit. 2014;33(4):311–3.
6. Lat A, Thompson GR 3rd. Update on the optimal use of voriconazole for invasive fungal infections. Infect Drug Resist. 2011;4:43–53.

8 Orbital Trauma and Reconstruction: A Case-Based Approach

Tarjani Vivek Dave and Akshita Agarwal

8.1 Case 1: Orbital Fracture with Adnexal Injury

A 23-year-old male was referred to our ophthalmic emergency unit following a motor vehicular accident. The patient had an episode of vomiting even prior to the examination could be attempted. There was an alleged history of a collision with a four-wheeler while the patient was riding his bike and a fall from the bike following the collision. The patient complained of a history of altered sensorium for a few minutes following the collision. He also complained of swelling over the eyes and the face, bleeding from the eyelid from a gaping wound, and diminution of vision in the left eye following trauma.

On examination, the right eye was within normal limits. The left upper eyelid had a partial thickness eyelid laceration involving the eyelid margin with exposed pre-aponeurotic fat (Fig. 8.1a) with surrounding eyelid edema and ecchymosis and a complete ptosis with orbital rim tenderness on palpation. There was a − 4 limitation of elevation with left hypoglobus (Fig. 8.1b). The vision in the left eye was PL PR inaccurate. There was subconjunctival chemosis, grade 3 RAPD, AC cells with Berlin's oedema in the inferior fundus, a 0.3 cup disc ratio, and the globe was intact with a normal digital tension.

Computed tomography of the orbit was suggestive of a left undisplaced fracture of the zygoma along with a fracture of the medial wall and the floor of the orbit. The inferior rectus muscle had prolapsed into the maxillary sinus, and there was a blow out floor fracture with a vertically oval configuration of the inferior rectus muscle.

A diagnosis of left multiple orbital wall fractures with traumatic optic neuropathy and an eyelid laceration involving the eyelid margin were made. On systemic examination, the patient continued to have bradycardia and vomiting. A

T. V. Dave (✉) · A. Agarwal
Hariram Motumal Nasta and Renu Hariram Nasta Ophthalmic Plastic Surgery Service, Kallam Anji Reddy Campus, L V Prasad Eye Institute, Hyderabad, Telangana, India

A. Gupta, P. Tahiliani (eds.), *Oculoplastic and Orbit Casebook*, Current Practices in Ophthalmology, https://doi.org/10.1007/978-981-97-0593-1_8

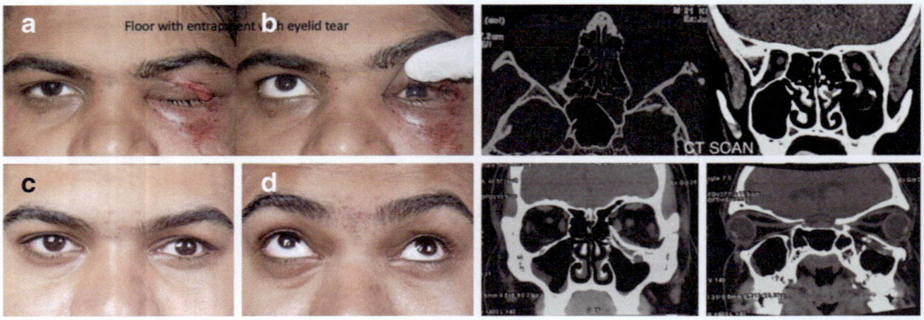

Fig. 8.1 Fracture of Orbital Floor with eyelid lacerations. (**a**) Complete eyelid ptosis with upper eyelid laceration, (**b**) Downward displaced eyeball with limitation in upgaze, (**c**) Postoperative 6 weeks shows a normal palpebral aperture with mild exotropia, (**d**) Postoperative 6 weeks shows recovery of upgaze movement in the left eye. CT scan: Shows pre and post fracture repair

confirmation of an oculo-cardiac reflex was made in consultation with the treating intensivist, and he was started on systemic anticholinergic drugs. He was promptly planned for repair of the eyelid laceration along with an orbitotomy for exploration and repair of the orbital floor and medial wall fracture. Inter-operatively the levator aponeurosis was found to be disinserted in the area beneath the eyelid tear, and it was anchored to the superior tarsus with a single 6-0 prolene suture to avoid post-operative ptosis. Upper eyelid tear was repaired with interrupted 6-0 vicryl sutures, and the eyelid margin was repaired with a vertical mattress silk suture. Inferior transconjunctival was incision taken and the orbital floor was explored. An inferior orbital floor fracture was noted infero-medial to the neurovascular bundle and with extension of fracture into the medial wall. Orbital fat and inferior rectus were found to be entrapped in the floor fracture. The posterior ledge of bone along the orbital floor was noted to be intact. All the entrapped soft tissue and fat were teased out of the fractured wall, and a prefabricated 3D titanium mesh was placed to correct the fracture. The titanium mesh was fixed with screws on the anterior surface of inferior orbital rim.

The patient was treated with iv antibiotics and methylprednisolone (in view of the traumatic optic neuropathy) in the postoperative period.

Six weeks following the trauma, the patient had 1 mm of relative enophthalmos on the left side, no ptosis, and good ocular motility; however, the vision remained suboptimal due to traumatic optic neuropathy (Fig. 8.1c and d). A repeat imaging was suggestive of a well-positioned 3D plate with good restoration of the orbital volume.

The learning

1. In the setting of acute trauma when there is an indication for repair of lacerations in the peri-orbital area, fracture repair should be combined.
2. An entrapped inferior rectus can lead to oculo-cardiac reflex in adults as well.
3. The presence of an oculo-cardiac reflex should necessitate an early repair of the fracture before the muscle goes into necrosis.

4. Exposed pre-septal fat should lead a surgeon to check the levator aponeurosis and if found to be disinserted the edge should be identified and reattached to the upper border of the tarsus.
5. Combined floor and medial wall fractures can be managed with a prefabricated titanium 3D mesh.

8.2 Case 2: Medial Wall and Floor Fracture Involving the Orbital Rim

A 37-year-old male presented to OPD with the complaints of blurring of vision in LE for the past 1 month following a road traffic accident 1 month ago. He gave a history of being diagnosed with fracture of maxillary bone for which maxillary bone fracture repair was done elsewhere 4 days after the injury.

On examination, right eye had subconjunctival haemorrhage; however, rest of the anterior segment was within normal limits. The left eye had subconjunctival haemorrhage with −1 restriction of extraocular movements. Enophthalmos of 3 mm was noted (Fig. 8.2). He had infraorbital nerve anaesthesia. The vision in the left eye was 20/40. There was resolving vitreous haemorrhage with traumatic optic neuropathy.

Computed tomography of the orbit was suggestive of left orbital floor with medial wall fracture involving the inferior orbital rim. A straight plate was seen holding the fragments of the comminuted rim fracture in place. The floor and medial wall fracture was large and involved the posteromedial strut. The posterior ledge was intact. The inferior rectus muscle was prolapsed in the maxillary sinus and was vertically elongated suggestive of a tug over the muscle sheath or the muscle. Medial wall fracture was small and was in the mid ethmoid region.

A diagnosis of left medial wall and floor fracture with traumatic optic neuropathy was made, and a repair with a prefabricated 3D titanium plate was performed. The fracture site was approached through inferior transconjunctival incision with a swinging eyelid approach. The incision was extended towards the caruncle to expose the medial wall of the orbit. Lateral canthotomy and cantholysis was done.

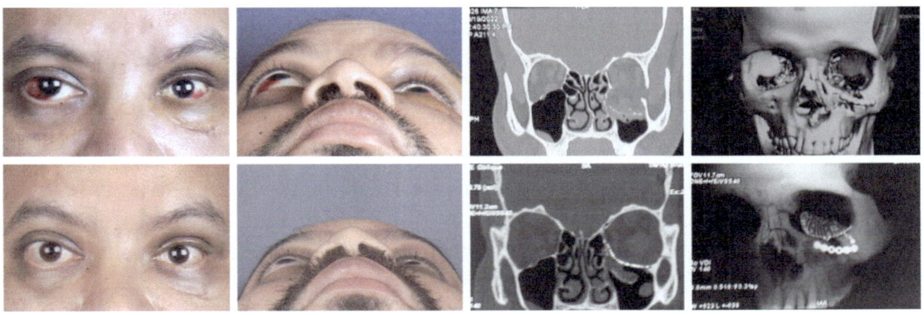

Fig. 8.2 Clinical picture and imaging showing enophthalmos

Inferior wall was exposed by hand-to-hand technique. The neovascular bundle was identified and protected throughout the procedure. Soft tissue was dissected out from the maxillary sinus into the orbit. Posterior maxillary wall was palpated and posterior ledge was identified. A prefabricated titanium 3D plate was inserted and placed such that the posterior end of the plate was in contact with the posterior ledge. The positioning of the plate on the medial wall was confirmed, and the foot-plate was secured to the inferior orbital rim with 4 mm self-tapping screws. The lateral canthus was reformed, and the conjunctival wounds secured with a couple of 6.0 vicryl sutures. Six weeks following the surgery, the patient had 2 mm of relative enophthalmos on the left side, no ptosis, and good ocular motility. A repeat imaging was suggestive of a well-positioned 3D plate with good restoration of the orbital volume.

The learning

1. When the posteromedial strut is involved in a fracture, placement of a barrier implant is not advisable since the implant will not have a 4-point support.
2. Despite adequate correction of the fracture, residual enophthalmos remains the most common complication.
3. This is due to the component of fat and soft tissue atrophy that is difficult to account for following trauma.
4. Raising the posterior end of the plate will help reduce the orbital volume and therefore help correct enophthalmos to an extent.

8.3 Case 3: White-Eyed Blow Out Fracture

A 9-year-old male child was referred to our ophthalmic emergency unit following trauma with glass table 2 days ago. Following the trauma, the child had three episodes of vomiting for the child complained of pain and diplopia on looking up.

On examination, the child was conscious and oriented. Bradycardia with a pulse rate was 46/min. Right eye was within normal limit. Left eye had extraocular motility restriction of −3 in upgaze. Rest of the left eye findings were unremarkable. An intravenous line was immediately secured, and the pulse rate was maintained with injection glycopyrrolate.

With a suspicion of muscle entrapment, an urgent CT scan was requested for. Serial computed tomography of the orbit showed entrapment of the inferior rectus muscle and the extraconal fat in the maxillary sinus with an intact orbital floor (Fig. 8.3).

A diagnosis of left white-eyed blow out orbital floor fracture with muscle entrapment was made. Intraoperatively, forced duction test was positive in upgaze. Inferior conjunctival incision was made with a radiofrequency cautery, and the floor of the orbit was exposed. Periosteal incision was made, and periosteum reflected on either side of the neurovascular bundle. Are area of crack in the bone was localised and an osteotomy performed to remove a segment of bone such the prolapsed orbital tissues could be repositioned in the orbit. Forced duction test was repeated to confirm

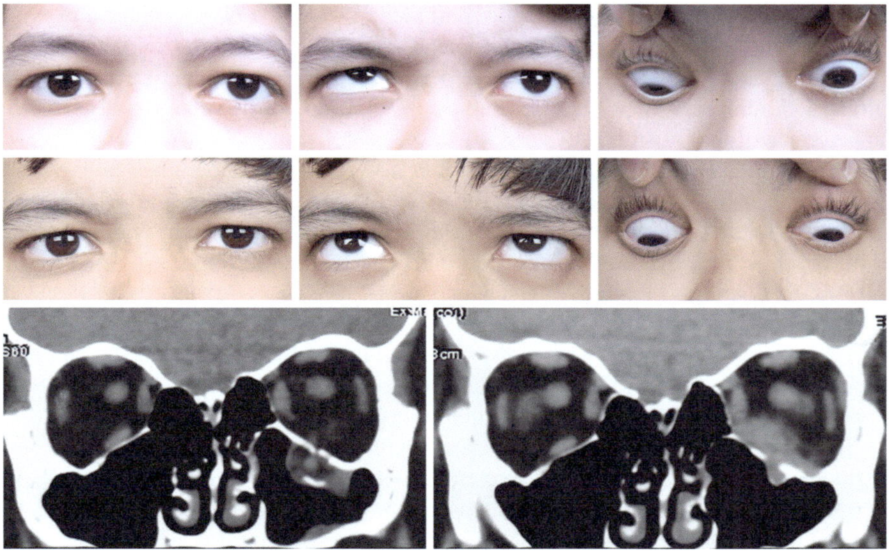

Fig. 8.3 Limitation of upgaze with entrapped muscle seen on CT scan

that there is no restriction of movement in upgaze. A polycaprolactone absorbable barrier implant placed to Conjunctiva was closed with single 6/0 polyglactin suture.

The patient was treated with iv antibiotics and methylprednisolone (in view of the traumatic optic neuropathy) in the postoperative period.

Six weeks following the surgery, the child had no enophthalmos ptosis or limitation of upgaze. A repeat imaging was suggestive of a well-positioned osteo-mesh.

The learning

1. Nausea and vomiting following trauma point towards head injury. However, when it is coupled with bradycardia, attention should be paid to rule out an oculo-cardiac reflex.
2. CT orbit in a case of a trap-door fracture will not demonstrate a fracture in the floor of the orbit. Careful review of sequential coronal cuts will demonstrate the inferior rectus muscle in the maxillary sinus.
3. In the presence of an oculo-cardiac reflex, early repair of orbital floor fracture is warranted.

8.4 Case 4: Orbital Fracture with Prosthetic Eye

A 19-year-old lady was referred for orbital reconstruction following a facial fracture repair and immediate trauma management elsewhere in 2014. She was using a prosthetic eye on the right side following the road traffic accident. A diagnosis of phthisis bulbi with fracture of the floor and medial wall of orbit was made and evisceration with polymethyl methacrylate implant of 20 mm diameter with floor fracture repair using a sialistic sheet was performed, and an ocular prosthesis was advised. Four years later, she presented with a complain of suboptimal aesthetic appearance of the prosthetic eye.

On examination, the right prosthetic had a hypotropic appearance; however, it was stable in the eye socket with a superior sulcus deformity and a lower eyelid retraction with the prosthetic eye in situ. She also had a significant enophthalmos with the prosthetic eye on the right side. The prosthetic eye weighed 3.5 g and was 10 mm in thickness. B scan was suggestive of a pre-phthisical eye with reduced axial length. Left eye was within normal limit.

Computed tomography was suggestive of a hypodense linear sialistic implant along the floor of the orbit with residual orbital volume expansion. A hyperdense spherical 20 mm implant was seen in the orbit (Fig. 8.4).

In view of the residual volume expansion in the orbit, the patient was advised right eye silicone sheet implant exchange with a porous. The surgery was performed via an inferior transconjunctival incision. The sialistic sheet was seen to have a tough capsule around it and was removed from the orbit after incising the capsule. All the orbital tissues were retracted, and a regular right porous polyethylene wedge implant was placed in the orbit. Good correction of enophthalmos was noted on table. The patient was dispensed with a prosthetic eye after 6 weeks following the placement of which the lower eyelid retraction completely resolved.

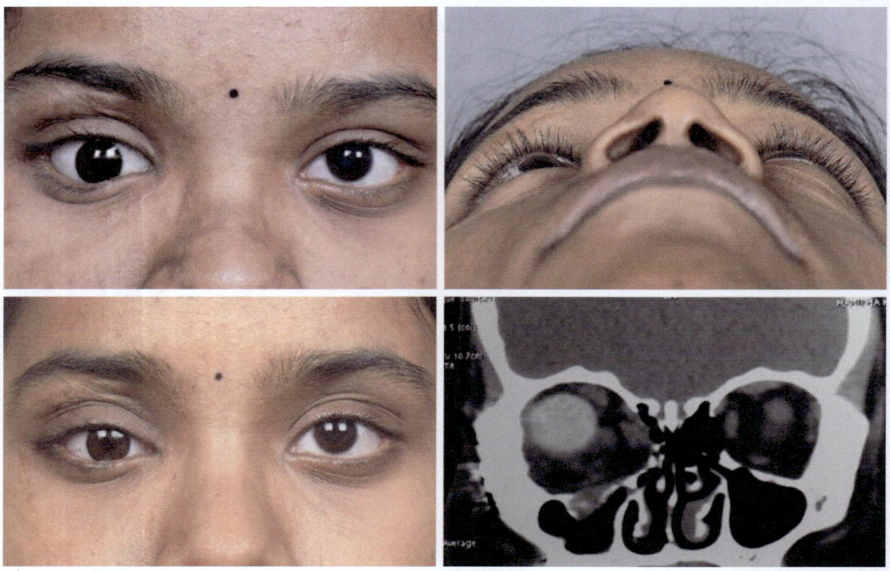

Fig. 8.4 Displaced prosthesis and migrated implant seen

The learning

1. Barrier sheets need the presence of a 4-point contact in the orbit for stability. This includes the infero-medial strut, the posterior ledge, and the anterior and lateral bony support.
2. If the infero-medial strut is displaced, the barrier sheet is likely to migrate towards the ethmoid sinus.
3. In an anophthalmic socket with a fracture, if the volume augmentation in the orbit is suboptimal, the prosthesis is generally larger and heavier resulting in a lower eyelid retraction.
4. Treatment of this eyelid retraction requires volume augmentation in the orbit and not an eyelid-tightening procedure.

8.5 Case 5: Displaced Lateral Wall Fracture Involving Zygoma

A 21-year-old male presented following a road traffic accident 5 months ago. The patient underwent a zygoma fracture repair elsewhere 4 days after the injury and was having double vision since then.

On examination, right eye findings were unremarkable. Left eye had severe ptosis with levator palpebrae superioris action of 5 mm and a grade 4 superior sulcus deformity and lateral canthal dystopia. There was hypoglobus with 3 mm of residual relative enophthalmos. Extraocular movements were restricted in elevation (−2) and abduction (−1) with diplopia in these gazes. Vision was 20/20, N6 in both eyes.

Computed tomography was suggestive of a three-wall orbital fracture involving the floor, medial wall, and the zygoma (Fig. 8.5). The zygoma was plated during the previous intervention at the frontozygomatic and the zygomatico-maxillary suture lines; however, the fracture had not been reduced adequately with a residual defect between two fragments of the zygoma (arrow) and inferior displacement of the lower fragment of the zygoma. Floor and medial wall were large with displacement of the infero-medial strut of the orbit and prolapse of the inferior rectus into the maxillary sinus.

A diagnosis of multiple orbital wall fractures was made, and patient was planned for secondary orbital reconstruction. Pre-existing cutaneous scars were used to approach the zygoma at the frontozygomatic (FZ) and the zygomatico-maxillary suture lines. The periosteum over the existing miniplates was incised, and the plates and screws were removed. Thick callus was noted over the intact portion of lateral wall of orbit, and the FZ plate was left in place. Caldwell-Luc incision was taken, and periosteum was elevated, and the maxillary plate and screws were removed. A malar osteotomy was performed to mobilise the inferior fragment of the zygoma. Open reduction and internal fixation were performed for the displaced fragment of the zygoma. The fragment was aligned with lateral wall and inferior orbital rim and area and fixed in place with miniplates and screws. Orbital floor dissection was performed after the periosteum was elevated to retrieve the orbital soft tissue prolapsed into the sinus. The posterior ledge was found to be deficient; a precontoured

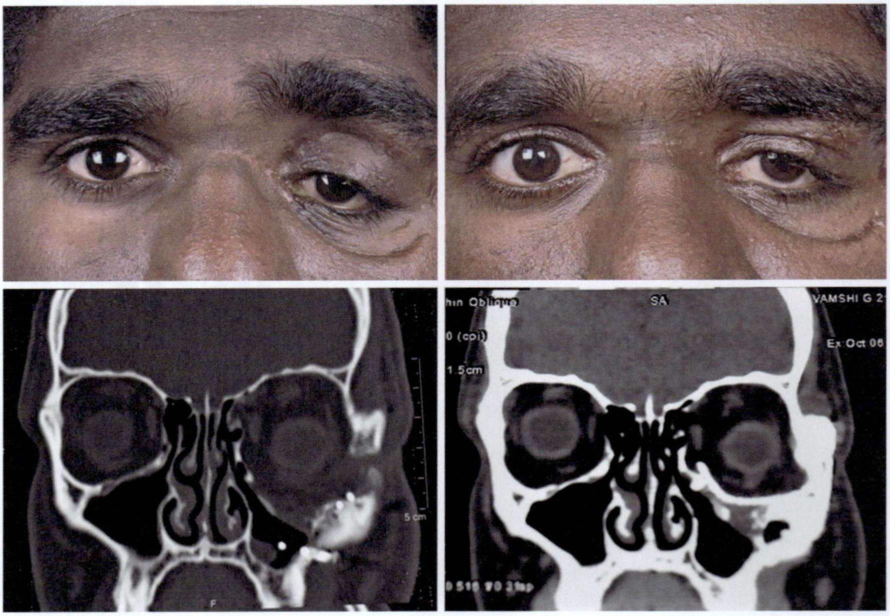

Fig. 8.5 Lateral canthal dystopia with displaced zygomatic bone

3D titanium mesh was placed in the orbit based on the inferior rim, and the foot plates of the mesh implant were fixed to the orbital rim with 4 mm screws. Adequate proptosis was achieved on table.

Six weeks postoperatively an improvement in the canthal dystopia, ptosis, enophthalmos, and the superior sulcus deformity were noted. A lateral droop in the upper eyelid was present. The extraocular movements were full and free. Two millimetre of left eye residual enophthalmos, with hypoglobus was noted. The patient was not keen for any further interventions and therefore was kept under observation. A postoperative CT orbit was suggestive of better reduction of the zygomatic fracture with a 3D titanium mesh implant in situ and minimal residual volume augmentation.

The learning

1. Lateral canthal dystopia is a clinical sign of a displaced zygoma.
2. Open reduction followed by internal fixation is the way to approach a zygomatic fracture.
3. A multidisciplinary team of an ophthalmic plastic surgeon with a maxillo-facial surgeon would be able to offer a better aesthetic outcome in complex fractures.

Financial Disclosures None.

Conflict of Interest None.

9 Orbital and Adnexal Tumors

Harshita Sharma and Sonal P. Yadav

9.1 Introduction

Orbital tumors or mass lesions are rare with an estimated incidence rate of 1.59 per million person-years, while lacrimal gland tumors occur at the estimated rate of 0.43 per million person-years [1]. Orbital and adnexal tumors can be classified in various ways. Depending on the etiopathology, there are six main types, namely, developmental, infectious, inflammatory, vascular, neoplastic, and miscellaneous; while depending on the cellular origin, they can be primary (originating from orbit including lacrimal gland), secondary (originating from surrounding structures as paranasal sinuses and involving orbit in contiguity, conjunctiva, lacrimal sac, middle cranial fossa, etc), and metastatic (disseminating from primary malignancy elsewhere). The signs and symptoms depend upon the etiology, location, and chronicity of the tumors. Proptosis, palpable mass lesion, ptosis, double vision, and occasionally pain can be the common presenting features. A thorough clinical evaluation and use of appropriate imaging technique and ancillary testing are essential to arrive at possible differential diagnosis. Histopathology is often required to finalize the diagnosis with the exception of vascular malformations where radiological imaging is relied upon for diagnosis. The surgical approach to an orbital mass for planned incision or excision biopsy depends upon the involved orbital space, dimension and extent of the tumor, relation with optic nerve and extraocular muscles, and involvement of adjacent soft tissues and bony destruction.

This chapter presents five cases involving orbital tumors. Each case discusses the clinical, radiological, and histopathological features of the respective tumor in detail.

H. Sharma · S. P. Yadav (✉)
Department of Ophthalmic Plastic Surgery, Orbit and Ocular Oncology, PBMA's H V Desai Eye Hospital, Pune, India
e-mail: sonal.yadav@hvdeh.org

A. Gupta, P. Tahiliani (eds.), *Oculoplastic and Orbit Casebook*, Current Practices in Ophthalmology, https://doi.org/10.1007/978-981-97-0593-1_9

9.2 Case 1—Cavernous Hemangioma of the Orbit

A 39-year-old gentleman presented to us with gradual, painless, and progressive protrusion of his left eye in the last 1 year. He had started noticing diminution of vision in left eye for the last 4 months. He denied any history of trauma or episodes of pain, redness, discharge in the eye. He did not notice any waxing or waning or diurnal variation in the amount of protrusion. He had no significant medical or surgical illness in the past.

On examination, left eye showed proptosis of 7 mm with superior dystopia of 4 mm (Fig. 9.1a and d). A firm non-compressible, non-reducible mass was palpable in the inferior quadrant with resistance to retropulsion. There was no change noted after Valsalva maneuver or postural variation. The best corrected visual acuity (BCVA) in right eye was 6/6, N6 and left eye was 6/12, N6. Anterior and posterior segment was unremarkable in right eye while left eye showed the presence of dilated conjunctival vessels in the inferior fornix along with normal anterior segment and choroidal folds in the posterior segment examination. Intraocular pressure in both

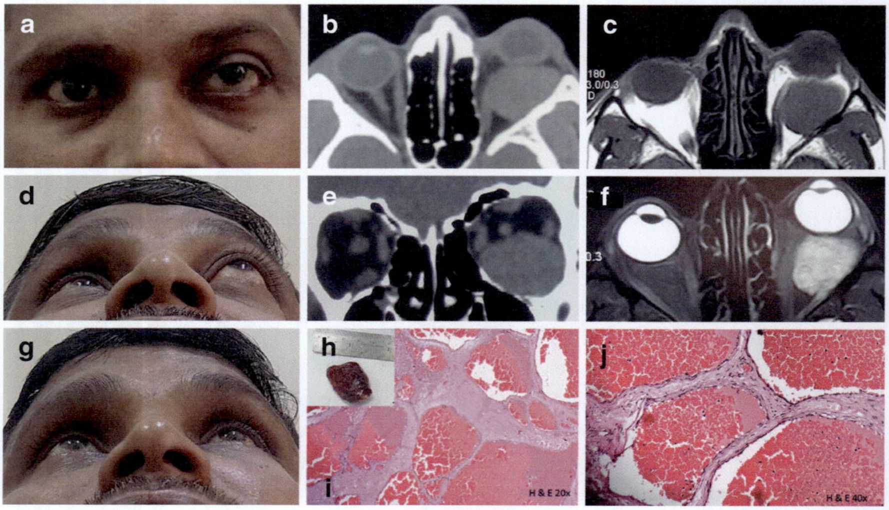

Fig. 9.1 Cavernous hemangioma of the orbit- 39/M, presenting with proptosis and superior dystopia in left eye, (**a** and **d**); CT scan-axial (**b**) and coronal (**e**) section shows well-circumscribed homogenous isodense (as compared to sclera) extraconal mass in the inferior quadrant, abutting the globe and causing scleral indentation. The inferior orbital wall showed thinning and excavation changes without evidence of bony erosion. MR imaging shows the tumor as hypointense on T1-weighted (**c**) and hyperintense on T2-weighted (**f**) images. The lesion appears purple-dark red on gross inspection (**h**) and microscopically, (**i, j**) it shows the presence of a vascular neoplasm composed of endothelial-lined spaces surrounded by a well-delineated fibrous capsule. Large cavernous vascular channels or spaces are seen separated by scant connective tissue stroma. Postoperatively, complete resolution of proptosis and dystopia without any cutaneous scar is appreciated (**g**)

eyes was within normal limits. Extraocular movements showed limitation of elevation and depression in left eye with rest of the gazes being full and free.

Computer tomography (CT) scan showed the presence of a 3.5 × 3 × 2.5 cm, well-circumscribed, homogenous isodense (as compared to sclera) intraconal mass lesion predominantly in the inferior quadrant, abutting the globe and causing scleral indentation. The inferior orbital wall showed thinning and excavation changes without evidence of bony erosion (Fig. 9.1b and e). Magnetic resonance imaging (MRI) of the orbit showed the lesion to be hypointense on T1-weighted scan and hyperintense on T2-weighted scan. Optic nerve was displaced medially and superiorly by the lesion (Fig. 9.1c and f).

He underwent transconjunctival orbitotomy with inferior forniceal approach and complete excision of the orbital tumor (Fig. 9.1h). Histopathological examination showed the presence of a vascular neoplasm composed of endothelial-lined spaces surrounded by a well-delineated fibrous capsule. Large cavernous vascular channels or spaces were seen separated by scant connective tissue stroma (Fig. 9.1i and j). The diagnosis of cavernous hemangioma was thus confirmed.

At 6-week postoperative follow-up, he showed complete resolution of proptosis (Fig. 9.1g), BCVA of 6/6, N6 with resolution of choroidal folds and full and free extraocular movements. At the last follow-up of 20 months, he continues to do well without any evidence of local recurrence.

9.2.1 Discussion

Cavernous hemangioma is the most common benign orbital tumor in adults comprising 3.1–9% of histopathologically proven tumors. On CT scan, they are seen as well- circumscribed round to oval lesions occupying intraconal (more common) or extraconal compartments. On MRI, the tumor is usually isointense to the cerebral gray matter or extraocular muscles on T1-weighted images (Fig 9.1c) and hyperintense on T2-weighted images (Fig 9.1f). On contrast injection, the lesion shows progressive filling and heterogenous enhancement. Complete surgical excision of the tumor is the treatment of choice. The surgical approach should be decided after consideration of size of the lesion, involved quadrant and its relationship with optic nerve and extraocular muscles. Careful blunt dissection should be carried out to free the lesion from surrounding orbital soft tissue. Cryoprobe can be applied to provide gentle traction while extracting the lesion after due dissection. Delayed recurrence in case of residual lesion in the orbit after an incomplete excision has been reported [2]. Asymptomatic tumors located in the posterior orbit can be observed and managed conservatively with close monitoring for signs of optic nerve compression and visual loss. Fractionated stereotactic radiotherapy has been used to effectively treat lesions located at orbital apex avoiding surgical morbidity and damage to optic nerve [3].

9.3 Case 2—External Angular Dermoid

A 3-year-old female child was brought by her mother after noticing gradual, painless, and progressive increase in the size of mass lesion on the outer corner of left eyebrow for the last 18 months. The antenatal and birth history was unremarkable. Her mother denied any history of trauma, episodes of pain, redness or discharge or diurnal and postural variation in the size of the lesion.

On examination, a soft to firm well-defined mass lesion was palpable along the superior orbital rim in the lateral quadrant, which was mobile, non-tender, noncompressible, and non-reducible (Fig. 9.2a). There was no change in the size of the lesion on crying or feeding or bending down. Overlying skin was normal. The lesion was found to be adherent to underlying periosteum at the lateral orbital rim. Best corrected visual acuity (BCVA) in Both eyes was 6/6, N6. Anterior segment and posterior segment examination was within normal limits. Computed Tomography (CT) scan showed the presence of a 1.8 × 1.3 × 0.6 cm in dimension, well-defined cystic mass lesion laterally along the superior orbital rim with no orbital extension (Fig. 9.2b). The features were suggestive of an external angular dermoid cyst. The child underwent anterior orbitotomy via eyelid crease approach with complete excision of the cyst followed by histopathology examination which revealed a well-encapsulated cyst with stratified squamous epithelium with the presence of hair follicles, sebaceous glands, and keratin (Fig. 9.2d and e). Intra- and postoperative recovery was uneventful and at

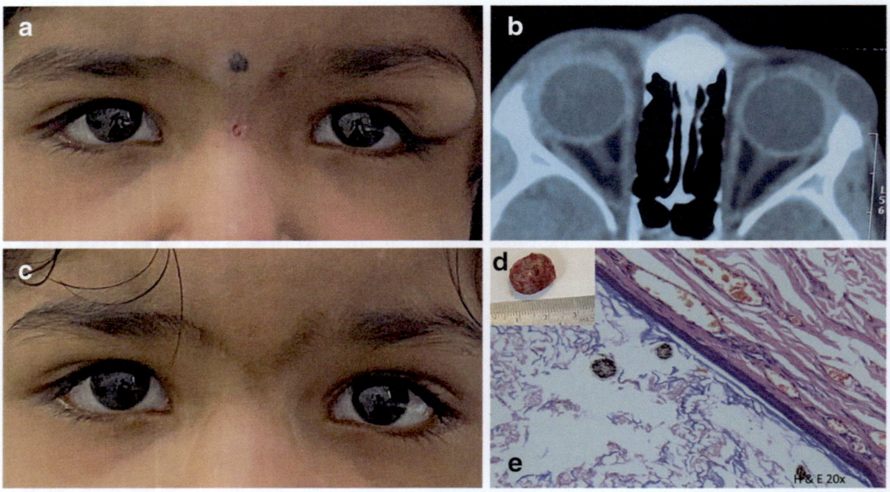

Fig. 9.2 External Angular Dermoid-3/F, presenting with localized soft lesion along lateral aspect of left eyelid (**a**). CT scan shows corresponding well-circumscribed cystic lesion with attachment to periosteum of lateral orbital rim without intra-orbital extension (**b**). On gross inspection, encapsulated oval pinkish cystic lesion is identified (**d**). Microscopically, (**e**) a wall lined by stratified squamous epithelium with lamellar flakes in the lumen with hair follicles is seen consisting with dermoid cyst. Postoperatively at follow-up of 1.5 months, the eyelid margin wound has healed well with good cosmetic outcome (**c**)

a follow-up of 6 weeks the child showed adequate wound healing with minimally visible and cosmetically acceptable eyelid scar (Fig. 9.2c).

9.3.1 Discussion

Dermoid cyst is a commonly found benign orbital tumor in pediatric age group. They are choristomas originating from the aberrant ectodermal tissue. During embryological development as the two suture lines of the skull close dermal or epidermal elements may be pinched off and form cysts, which are adjacent to the suture line. Most common sites of occurrence are frontozygomatic and frontolacrimal sutures. Depending on the site of origin, they can be classified as: sutural, anterior orbital, deep orbital, trans-orbital, intraosseous, or conjunctival.

The presenting clinical features include palpable mass in the orbit, proptosis, dystopia, pain or oscillopsia on chewing, etc. Ruptured or leaking dermoid cyst may present with signs of preseptal or orbital inflammation. External angular location is most common for an anterior orbital dermoid. They can present with periosteal attachment or attachment to frontozygomatic suture. Histopathologically, dermoids contain desquamated squamous epithelium and keratin in the lumen and are encapsulated while lined by keratinized stratified squamous epithelium. Hair follicles, sweat glands, apocrine glands as well as lacrimal gland may also appear in the cyst wall.

Complete surgical excision is the treatment of choice for a dermoid. Inflammation, recurrence, and fistula can complicate capsular breach and incomplete excision. Hence, the emphasis is provided on complete excision.

9.4 Case 3—Diffuse Orbital Lymphangioma

A 34-year-old lady sought consult for noticing gradual, progressive protrusion of her right eye for last 4 years. The protrusion was associated with occasional dull-aching pain and strain in the right eye. She denied any history of trauma, double vision, or decrease in vision in that eye. She reported having diminished vision in her left eye and was diagnosed case of amblyopia as per past records.

On examination, her BCVA in right eye was 6/6, N6 and left eye was 6/60, N24. She had axial proptosis of 5 mm in the right eye and showed no change on Valsalva maneuver or lying down position (Fig. 9.3a and b). Slight increase in retrobulbar resistance was noted but no palpable thrill or bruit was appreciated. Extraocular movements were full and free in all direction of gazes. Rest of anterior segment and fundus examination of right eye was withing normal limits. Left eye examination was unremarkable.

CT scan of the orbit revealed an ill-defined heterogenous iso-hypodense infiltrating mass lesion in superomedial quadrant with mulberry like appearing cysts involving both extraconal and intraconal compartments with few hyperdense phleboliths (Fig. 9.3d and e). The lesion was noted in close proximity with superior

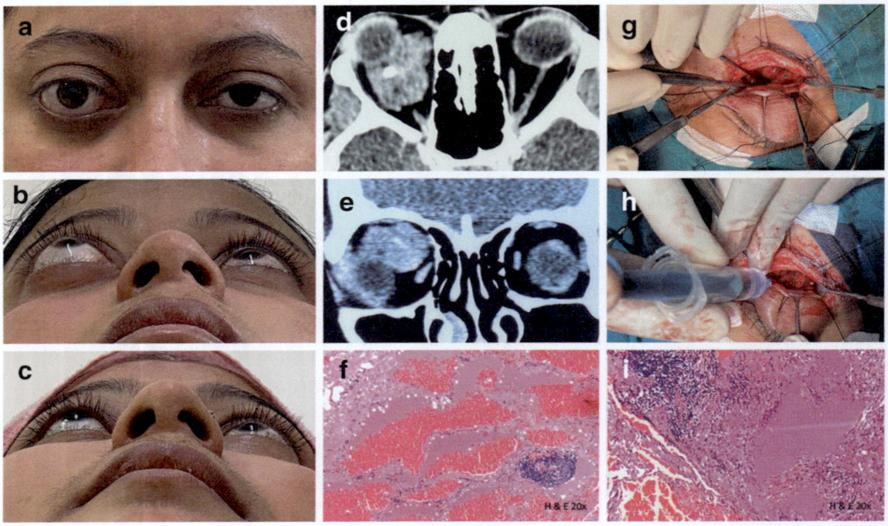

Fig. 9.3 Diffuse lymphangioma of the orbit- 39/F presented with axial proptosis of right eye, (**a** and **b**) with CT scan on axial (**d**) and coronal (**e**) sections showing ill-defined iso-hyperdense mass lesion in both extraconal and intraconal compartment with the presence of phleboliths in superior-medial quadrant of right orbit. Intraoperatively, lesion appears as thin-walled fluid-filled cystic mass (**g**). Surgical debulking was carried out along with intralesional sclerotherapy with Injection Bleomycin to the residual lesion (**h**). Microscopically, the neoplasm contains dilated lymphovascular channels with lymphatic and RBCs in lumen (**f**) and hyperplastic lymphoid follicles in interstitium (**i**) suggestive of lympho-venous malformation (lymphangioma) with secondary hemorrhage. Postoperatively at 18 months of follow-up, she shows good regression in the amount of proptosis (**c**) without evidence of secondary hemorrhage or recurrence

rectus-levator palpebrae superioris complex, and it was displacing the optic nerve infero-laterally. The features were suggestive of a diffuse orbital lymphangioma.

She underwent lateral orbitotomy with sub-brow approach with debulking the lesion and intralesional sclerotherapy with injection Bleomycin (5 U/mL) (Fig. 9.3g and h). Early postoperative period was uneventful.

The gross examination of debulked specimen showed a brownish gray soft lesion, and microscopically it had cystically dilated endothelium lined spaces containing eosinophilic proteinaceous material and intraluminal RBCs and lymphoplasmacytic infiltrated stroma (Fig. 9.3f and i). The findings were consistent with the diagnosis of orbital lymphangioma with secondary hemorrhage. She showed resolution of proptosis and good bilateral symmetry with mild aponeurotic ptosis postoperatively (Fig. 9.3c). The pre-operative BCVA and extraocular movements status was unchanged. At the last follow-up of 18 months, she continues to do well without any evidence of local recurrence.

9.4.1 Discussion

Orbital Lymphangiomas are benign lymphatic hamartomatous lesions appearing as multi-cystic localized malformations involving lymphatic and vascular systems. They are commonly encountered in the head and neck region in the first and second decade of life. Lymphangiomas are classified as no-flow (Type 1) malformations as per the blood flow type; veno-lymphatic or lympho-venous malformation as per the predominant vascular system involvement and microcystic (cysts <2 cm) and macrocystic (cysts >2 cm) and mixed depending upon the size of the cysts. They commonly present with slowly progressive proptosis, displacement of the globe, ptosis, and restriction of eye movements and in some cases with signs of spontaneous intra-orbital hemorrhage. In rare instances, compressive optic neuropathy and exposure keratopathy are encountered after sudden increase in proptosis due to intra-orbital hemorrhage. CT scan usually shows cyst-like lesions with mulberry appearance with variable contrast enhancement. Cyst walls tend to show rim enhancement in cases with intra-cystic hemorrhage. On MRI, they are seen as isointense on T1-weighted images and hyperintense on T2 images, often with a presence of internal septations within the lesion. The characteristic findings include multiple cysts with air-fluid levels.

Management options include:

(a) Observation with serial imaging for patients without vision threatening symptoms or significant physical disfigurement.
(b) Intralesional sclerotherapy- Sclerotherapy with varied sclerosants like OK-432, sodium tetra-decyl sulfate, bleomycin, and doxycycline have been utilized for macrocystic lymphangiomas for effective lesion regression without significant long-term side effects. However they have been proven less effective for microcystic lymphangiomas in comparison to predominatly macrocystic type. Reported adverse effects of these agents include infection, bleeding, damage of adjacent structures during injection, and post-injection reactive inflammation.
(c) Medical therapy- Systemic Sildenafil (PDE-5 inhibitor) and Sirolimus (mTOR inhibitor) have been tried as measures to decrease the volume of microcystic lesions with limited evidence.
(d) Surgery- Surgical excision or debulking of the lesion can be considered for selected cases. The surgical intervention is often challenging due to the infiltrative nature of the lesion, intraoperative risk of bleeding, residual lesion, and recurrence. In our experience, a combined approach where the predominantly microcystic component is surgical excised and residual or macrocystic component is given intralesional sclerotherapy has worked well with acceptable cosmetic outcome. The intralesional sclerotherapy can be repeated as indicated after 6–8 weeks interval till satisfactory regression is achieved.

9.5 Case 4—Pleomorphic Adenoma of Lacrimal Gland

A 31-year-old gentleman presented after noticing gradual progressive protrusion of left eye for last 8 months. There was no history of trauma, pain, double vision, or decrease in vision. There was no history of noticing any diurnal or postural variation. He had no significant medical or surgical illness in the past.

On examination, he showed proptosis of 2 mm with downward and nasal displacement of the globe (Fig. 9.4a and b). A firm mass with smooth surface was palpable along the superior orbital rim in the superolateral quadrant, and it was immobile, non-tender, non-compressible, and non-reducible. The lesion was in close proximity with the bony orbital rim and overlying skin was normal. Best corrected visual acuity (BCVA) in both eyes was 6/6, N6. Anterior segment and posterior segment examination and intraocular pressure was within normal limit for both eyes. The tear function as evaluated by Schirmer's test I was within normal limits and was bilaterally symmetrical.

Computed Tomography (CT) scan showed the presence of a 2.7 × 1.5 × 1.5 cm, oval and well-circumscribed isodense mass in the extraconal space in the superolateral quadrant extending from anterior to mid orbit (Fig. 9.4d and e). Mass was in

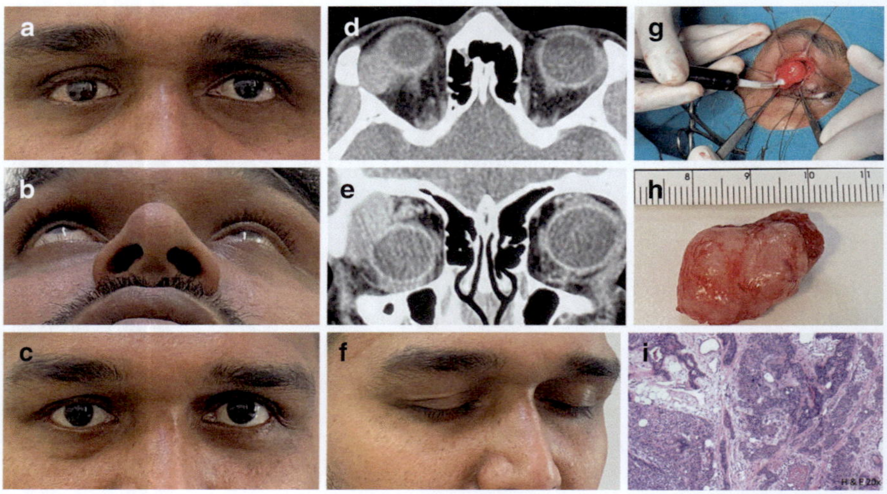

Fig. 9.4 Pleomorphic Adenoma of Lacrimal Gland-31/M shows mild proptosis and inferior displacement of right eye (**a** and **b**) with CT scan on axial (**d**) and coronal (**e**) section showing a well-circumscribed mass lesion in superior-temporal quadrant of right eye abutting the eyeball and causing its downward displacement. An eyelid crease approach orbitotomy was performed, and the lesion was completely excised with help of a cryoprobe (**g**). On gross inspection, it was pinkish white appearing smooth surfaced solid mass (**h**) and microscopically showed (**i**), well-encapsulated tumor composed of sheets of round and polygonal cells with clear cells. Epithelial component comprising tubules and cords lined with epithelial and myo-epithelial cells were also noted suggestive of pleomorphic adenoma of lacrimal gland. At 18 months of follow-up, he is doing well without any evidence of local recurrence (**c**) and minimally visible cosmetically acceptable eyelid crease scar (**f**)

close relation with superior rectus, superior oblique, and lateral rectus. Lacrimal gland could not be visualized separately from the lesion. No evidence of bony erosion was seen. The features were suggestive of a benign lacrimal gland tumor. He underwent lateral orbitotomy via an eyelid crease approach and cryoprobe-assisted excision of the mass (Fig. 9.4g) in toto followed by histopathology evaluation.

Gross examination showed a solid firm mass measuring 2.4 × 1.7 × 1.2 cm (Fig. 9.4h) and microscopically showed well-encapsulated tumor composed of sheets of round and polygonal cells with clear cells. Epithelial component comprising tubules and cords lined with epithelial and myo-epithelial cells were also noted. There was no evidence of atypia or invasive malignancy suggestive. The findings were consistent with diagnosis of pleomorphic adenoma of lacrimal gland. Postoperative recovery was uneventful and at a follow-up of 18 months, he continues to do well with good cosmesis and a minimal scar (Fig. 9.4c and i), without any functional deficit and shows no signs of recurrence.

9.5.1 Discussion

Pleomorphic adenoma is the most common benign neoplasm of lacrimal gland. Painless, progressive proptosis with downward and nasal displacement of the eye is the common presenting feature. On CT, they appear as round to oval well-circumscribed lesions with smooth surface causing displacement of the globe. Long-standing lesions may lead to bony excavation changes; however, bony erosions are uncommon. MRI imaging shows the tumor as hypointense on T1-weighted image and hyperintense on T2-weighted image. Complete surgical excision of the tumor is the treatment of choice. Incomplete excision or an incision biopsy is avoided in cases with pleomorphic adenoma as the 5-years recurrence rate at such instances has been recorded as >30%. In addition, recurrent pleomorphic adenoma can undergo malignant changes [4]. Thus, it is essential to clinically suspect these tumors prior to surgery to avoid inadvertent incision biopsy and ensure a complete surgical excision to reduce recurrence.

9.6 Case 5—Adenoid Cystic Carcinoma of Lacrimal Gland

A 23-year-old female presented with complains of gradual and progressive downward displacement of right eye for last 12 months. She had noticed tingling and dull-aching pain around her right periocular region, forehead and temporal fossa region, and gradually worsening double vision since last 6 months. She informed us of a history of similar complaints and had undergone excision by transcranial approach elsewhere 3 years back. However, surgical records or histopathology record from that time were not available. She denied history of any significant medical illness in the past and had not noticed significant change in her weight or appetite.

On examination, her best corrected visual acuity (BCVA) in right eye was 6/18, N12, and left eye was 6/6, N6. Right eye showed 4 mm of proptosis with 6 mm of inferior dystopia (Fig. 9.5a and b) with restricted extraocular movements in up-gaze resulting in diplopia. On palpation a firm, mildly tender mass was present along the superior orbital rim in superior orbit. The mass was non-compressible, and non-reducible. Superior orbital rim was irregular on palpation and overlying skin appeared normal. Anterior segment of right eye was normal. Dilated fundus examination showed choroidal folds in superior and temporal quadrants. Left eye examination was unremarkable.

CT scan showed a fairly well-defined hyperdense heterogenous mass in the superolateral quadrant extending from preseptal region to posterior orbit on the right side (Fig. 9.5d and e). The lesion was displacing the globe downwards. Superior rectus-levator palpebrae superioris (SR-LPS) complex and lateral rectus muscle were not seen separately from the lesion. Lacrimal gland could not be visualized separately from the lesion. Bony erosion was seen along superior orbital rim. Recurrent lacrimal gland tumor was suspected. She underwent lateral orbitotomy with sub-brow approach with en-bloc excision of the mass. Intraoperatively significant bony erosion along superior orbital rim was noted (Fig. 9.5g). The involved

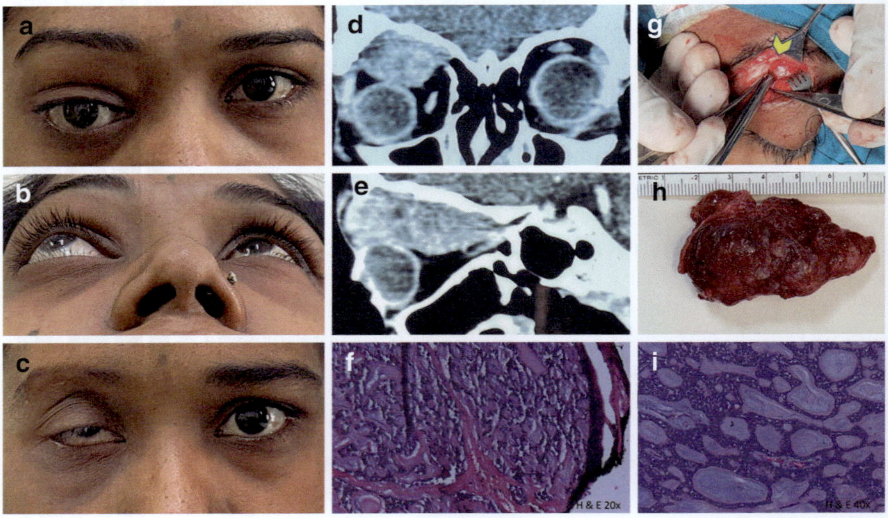

Fig. 9.5 Adenoid Cystic Carcinoma (AdCCa) of lacrimal gland-23/F presented with eccentric proptosis and inferior dystopia of right eye (**a** and **b**) with CT scan on axial (**d**) and sagittal (**e**) section showing an ill-defined heterogenous mass lesion in superior and temporal quadrant displacing the eyeball inferiorly and causing bony erosion along superior orbital rim possibly arising from lacrimal gland. Intraoperatively (**g**) significant bony destruction along superior orbital rim was visible (yellow arrowhead). On gross inspection of the mass, it was a solid lesion and had an irregular surface (**h**) and microscopically showed large, circumscribed nodules as well as infiltrating nests of basaloid cells arranged in tubular and cribriform pattern (**f** and **i**), the features suggestive of cribriform variety of AdCCa of lacrimal gland. At 15 months follow-up of surgery and adjuvant radiation, she is doing well with moderate ptosis (**c**) without any signs of local recurrence or systemic metastasis.

part of SR-LPS complex was excised along with the mass. Intraoperative and early postoperative period was uneventful.

Gross examination showed a solid grayish white firm mass measuring 6 × 3.4 × 1.6 cm (Fig. 9.5h). Microscopically, the tumor was composed of large, circumscribed nodules as well as infiltrating nests of basaloid cells arranged in tubular and cribriform pattern (Fig. 9.5f and i). The tumor cells had small, irregular hyperchromatic nuclei and scanty cytoplasm with focal areas of necrosis and focal perineural invasion was seen. Lymphovascular invasion was not identified. The above histopathological features were consistent with cribriform pattern of adenoid cystic carcinoma of lacrimal gland.

Postoperatively, she had moderate ptosis with residual restriction on elevation as a result of resection of involved SR-LPS muscle complex. She underwent systemic whole-body PET-CT scan to rule out systemic metastasis. She then received adjuvant radiotherapy (50 Gy in 28 fractions) with globe sparing intensity modulated radiotherapy technique. She denied adjuvant chemotherapy. She is under regular follow-up for clinical evaluation and imaging (CT scan of orbit at 6 months to look for local recurrence and whole-body PET scan yearly to look for systemic metastasis). At the last visit, 15 months since the completion of radiation, she is doing well with moderate ptosis in right eye and no evidence of local recurrence or systemic metastasis. (Fig. 9.5c).

9.6.1 Discussion

Adenoid cystic carcinoma (AdCCa) of lacrimal gland is the second most common epithelial tumor and the most common malignant epithelial tumor of lacrimal gland. AdCCa typically presents in the fourth and fifth decade of life, however, has been reported in children and elderly [5]. Clinically, it presents as slow to insidious onset mass lesion in superior-temporal quadrant with signs of palpable mass, globe displacement, ptosis, and diplopia. Pain and paresthesia are commonly associated due to the tumor's tendency of perineural invasion. On CT, the tumor appears as solid mass lesion with irregular margins and nodularity with adjacent soft tissue infiltration and bony destruction. MR imaging is helpful in assessing possible perineural invasion and extension into cavernous sinus and brain. The tumor appears isointense to muscles on both T1- and T2-weighted images with moderate contrast enhancement (?).

Treatment of AdCCa is challenging and common consensus on most effective modalities of treatment is yet to be reached due to rarity of the disease. The current management involves surgical tumor excision and adjuvant radiotherapy [6]. Surgical technique depends upon the tumor extent (bony involvement, perineural spread, intracranial involvement) and includes local excision, en-bloc removal, orbital exenteration, and radical exenteration. Although resection can be successful at achieving local and regional control, it has not reduced the incidence of distant metastases. Intra-arterial chemotherapy, adjuvant interstitial brachytherapy has been tried with limited evidence [7, 8].

Histopathologically, five morphological variants have been reported, namely, cribriform, basaloid, sclerosing, comedocarcinomatous, and tubular. Better prognosis is associated with cribriform variant while basaloid is associated with worst prognosis.

Local as well as systemic prognosis remains grave for those diagnosed with AdCCa of the lacrimal gland. Overall, 10-year survival rate was found to be between 20 and 40%. Mortality associated is typically due to intracranial spread or distant metastases. In addition to the brain, metastatic disease has been found in the lung, bone, liver, muscle, and spleen.

Acknowledgments The authors would like to acknowledge contributions from Nanda Kachare MD, Head of the Department of Histopathology and Cytology and Aniruddha Puntambekar MD, Consultant, Department of Histopathology at Ruby Hall Clinic, Pune for the histopathology images used in the chapter.

References

1. Hassan WM, Bakry MS, Hassan HM, Alfaar AS. Incidence of orbital, conjunctival and lacrimal gland malignant tumors in USA from surveillance, epidemiology and end results, 1973–2009. Int J Ophthalmol. 2016;9(12):1808–13.
2. Henderson JW, Farrow GM, Garrity JA. Clinical course of an incompletely removed cavernous hemangioma of the orbit. Ophthalmology. 1990;97:625–8.
3. Ratnayake GS, McNab AA, Dally MJ, Zajarski C, Senthi S, Ruben JD. Fractionated stereotactic radiotherapy for cavernous venous malformations of the orbital apex. Ophthalmic Plast Reconstr Surg. 2019;35(4):322–5.
4. Font RL, Gamel JW. Epithelial tumors of the lacrimal gland: an analysis of 265 cases. In: Jacobiec FA, editor. Ocular and adnexal tumors. Birmingham: Aesculapius Publishing; 1978. p. 787–805.
5. Andreoli MT, Aakalu V, Setabutr P. Epidemiological trends in malignant lacrimal gland tumors. Otolaryngol Head Neck Surg. 2015;152(2):279–83.
6. Esmaeli B, Golio D, Kies M, DeMonte F. Surgical management of locally advanced adenoid cystic carcinoma of the lacrimal gland. Ophthal Plast Reconstr Surg. 2006;22(5):366–70.
7. Tse DT. Clinical and microdissection genotyping analyses of the effect of intra-arterial cytoreductive chemotherapy in the treatment of lacrimal gland adenoid cystic carcinoma. Trans Am Ophthalmol Soc. 2005;103:337–67.
8. Shields JA, Shields CL, Freire JE, Brady LW, Komarnicky L. Plaque radiotherapy for selected orbital malignancies: preliminary observations: the 2002 Montgomery Lecture, part 2. Ophthal Plast Reconstr Surg. 2003;19(2):91–5.

10 Eyelid Malignant Tumors

Prerana Tahiliani and Adit Gupta

Eyelid tumors comprise 10–12% of all the skin cancers. The eyelid is composed of two lamellae, and malignancies may arise from either of these. Depending on the cell of origin, eyelid malignancies can be subclassified further. Clinically, malignant eyelid tumors may have one or more of the following signs:

1. Loss of eyelashes
2. Ulceration of skin.
3. Change in eyelid margin architecture.
4. Distortion of meibomian glands.
5. Feeder vessels and telangiectasia.
6. Sudden growth of lesion.
7. Irregular margins.

In this chapter, we will discuss the three commonly encountered eyelid malignancies.

10.1 Case 1: Sebaceous Gland Carcinoma

Sebaceous gland carcinoma is highly malignant, and potentially lethal tumor of the eyelid skin. The neoplasm arises from sebaceous glands, such as those of the meibomian glands in the tarsus, the Zeis glands of the eyelashes and rarely the caruncle, the glands in the periocular skin or eyebrow follicles. The lesion occurs more often

P. Tahiliani (✉)
Mumbai Eye Plastic Surgery, Mumbai, India

Lotus Eye Hospital, Mumbai, India

A. Gupta
Mumbai Eye Plastic Surgery, Mumbai, India

A. Gupta, P. Tahiliani (eds.), *Oculoplastic and Orbit Casebook*, Current Practices in Ophthalmology, https://doi.org/10.1007/978-981-97-0593-1_10

in the upper eyelid followed by the lower eyelid. It is one of the commonest eyelid malignancies in the Asian and Indian population.

10.1.1 Case Summary

A 60-year-male presented with a lower eyelid swelling since 6 months. This lesion was treated as a stye by a general ophthalmologist. There was no response to conservative management, and he underwent incision curettage of the lesion elsewhere. He was then referred for further management. Examination showed a nodular, yellowish white nodular lesion at the eyelid margin involving the tarsus and the meibomian glands. There was localized distortion of the tarsus with loss of eyelashes. No ulceration or bleeding was noted. Incision biopsy was performed which confirmed sebaceous gland carcinoma of the eyelid. He underwent systemic screening which revealed no metastasis. He then underwent eyelid tumor excision with 4 mm margins under frozen section control and edge cryotherapy. Eyelid reconstruction was performed in the same sitting using a Tenzel flap and mobilizing the lateral eyelid skin. He was recurrence free with a good cosmetic and functional outcome at 2 years.

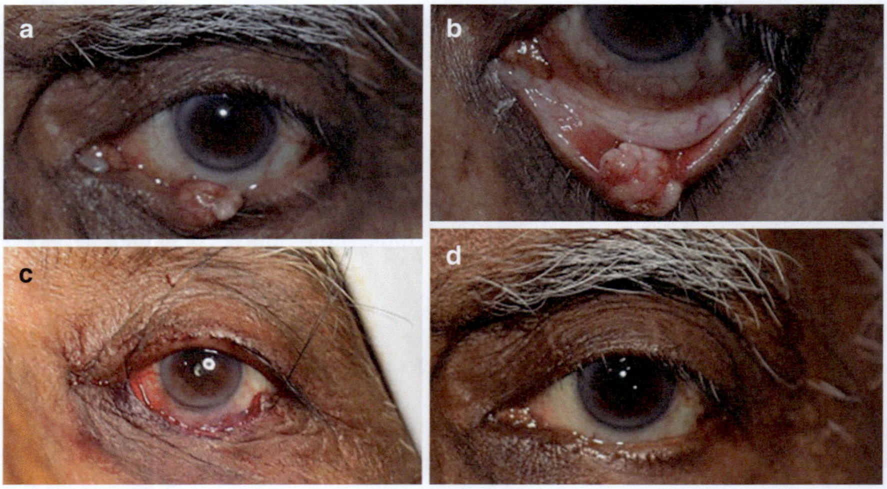

Case 1: (**a** and **b**) Image showing yellowish nodulo-ulcerative lesion on the lower eyelid, (**c**) Intraoperative image after excising the lesion with wide local margins, (**d**) 6-month postoperative picture after eyelid reconstruction surgery with no recurrence

10.1.2 Discussion

Sebaceous gland carcinoma (SGC) is commoner than basal cell carcinoma in the Asian and Indian subcontinent. It is a malignant tumor with propensity for systemic spread if not detected on time. The tumour can present as a mass as described or can occasionally masquerade as:

(a) Recurrent chalazion.
(b) Chronic blepharoconjunctivitis with red eye.

A high index of suspicion should be maintained in the above situations, and a biopsy should be performed in case of doubt.

The mass is usually painless and yellowish in color due to the presence of lipid within the cells.

It arises in the sebaceous gland and can extend up to the palpebral conjunctiva. Rarely, it can also arise from the sebaceous glands in the caruncle. Eversion of the eyelid is very important as sometimes a posterior early mass may be missed on primary cursory examination.

A hallmark of sebaceous gland carcinomas is "pagetoid spread"—spreading of tumor cells along the epithelium away from the main tumor. A map biopsy of sites away from the main mass can rule out skip lesions.

The mainstay of management is surgical excision with a wide margin of tumour free clearance during surgery. Intraoperative frozen section analysis and cryotherapy to the margins helps reduce local recurrence of the tumor. It is paramount to ensure a full-thickness specimen and obtain map biopsies of the conjunctiva where relevant. If the tumour invades into the orbit, orbital exenteration may be indicated for large orbital extensions. Staging is assessed using the TNM definitions as provided by the American Joint Committee on Cancer Recommendations (AJCC 8). Over the past decade neoadjuvant chemotherapy has shown promise in some advanced tumors to downsize the lesion followed by surgical excision. This has helped salvage the eyeball and vital structures in some cases with early orbital spread.

Factors that have been associated with a worse prognosis include

1. Localized or distant metastasis.
2. Orbital invasion.
3. Multicentric origin.
4. Poor differentiation on histopathology.
5. Tumor diameter exceeding 10 mm.
6. Pagetoid invasion.

SGC can recur in 33% of cases with metastasis rate of almost 20–25%. Systemic screening for distant metastasis and lymph node involvement is mandatory in all cases of SGC.

It is important for clinicians to be familiar with the varied presentations of sebaceous carcinoma of the eyelid so that patients receive prompt diagnosis and treatment of a potentially fatal disease.

10.2 Case 2: Basal Cell Carcinoma

Basal cell carcinoma (BCC), formerly also called rodent ulcer is a locally infiltrating carcinoma seen more commonly in the sun exposed areas of the body. It is commonly seen around the periocular area and is common in Caucasians. It is the most common eyelid malignancy worldwide. It generally grows slowly, invades local tissues, and rarely metastasizes.

10.2.1 Case Summary

A 65-year-old female with history of lower eyelid lesion was referred for treatment. She had a pigmented lesion on her left lower eyelid with area of central ulceration and rolled out margins. Additionally the lesion had an amelanotic component creeping over the eyelid margin. There was no evidence of regional lymphadenopathy and systemic examination was normal. Incision biopsy revealed a basal cell carcinoma. She then underwent wide local excision, margin cryotherapy, and eyelid reconstruction (Hughes flap from the upper eyelid and monopedicle skin flap for skin). There is no recurrence at 2-year follow-up.

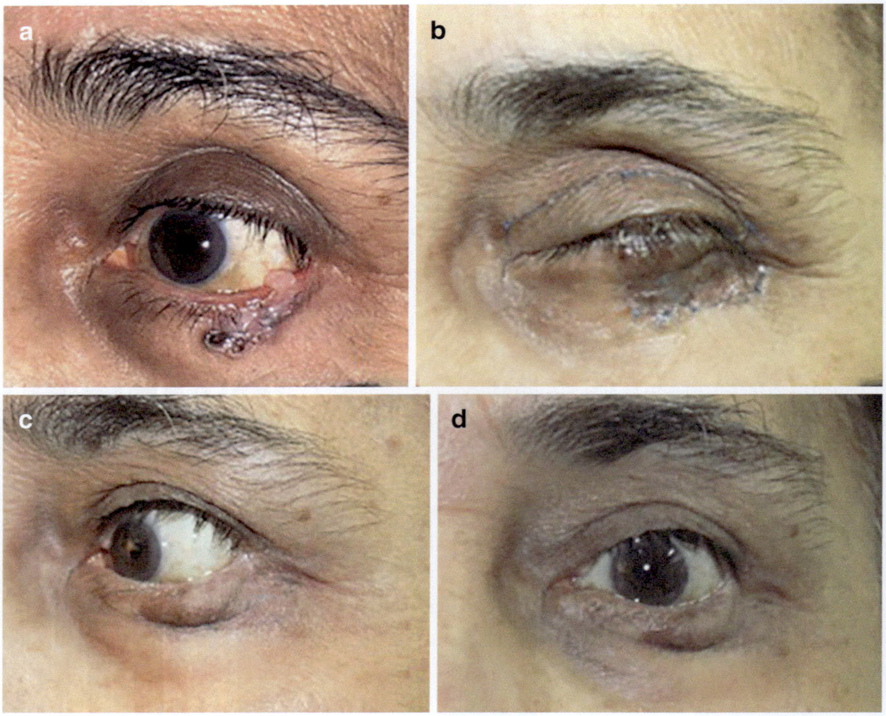

Case 2: (**a**) Lower eyelid ulcerated pigmented lesion seen extending up to the eyelid margin; (**b**) Post eyelid excision and reconstruction showing skin graft and monopedicle flap in place; (**c** and **d**) postoperative outcome showing mild eyelid retraction and bulk of the flap but no recurrence of tumor at 6 months

10.2.2 Discussion

Basal cell carcinoma is the commonest eyelid malignancy and is responsible for more than 60–70% of all eyelid tumors. The biggest risk factor for developing BCC is ultraviolet light exposure. Other risk factors include immunosuppression, fair skin, radiation exposure, syndromes like xeroderma pigmentosum. BCC occurs most frequently on the lower eyelid followed by medial canthus, upper eyelid, and lateral canthus. Clinically, it may appear like a nodulo-ulcerative lesion with rolled out edges. The various morphological types are: Superficial, nodular, and ulcerative. Nodular variety of BCC is the commonest morphological presentation. It presents as a pink, pearly papule with telangiectasia and rolled out edges. Another variant, morpheaform or superficial sclerosing, presents like a superficial scar and spreads superficially.

Surgical excision with wide margins (4 mm) is the gold standard for BCC treatment. Mohs surgery can be used to reduce the recurrence rate while excision. Excision under frozen section control is an option where Mohs surgery is not available. The above techniques help reduce the chances of recurrence after the primary surgery.

Topical imiquimod 5% and 5-Fluouracil creams have been used as an option for superficial lesions and in patients unfit for surgery. These topical formulations require application over multiple weeks. Vismodegib, a sonic hedgehog inhibitor was approved by the US FDA for locally advanced and metastatic BCC. The disadvantage of Vismodegib is the limited availability and cost of the drug. Radiation therapy also has been tried as an alternative in surgically unfit patients, recurrent disease, advanced tumors for palliative care.

The prognosis of BCC is excellent and if diagnosed early, surgical excision can provide a definitive cure for this malignancy.

10.3 Case 3: Squamous Cell Carcinoma

Squamous cell carcinoma (SCC) is a malignant tumor arising from the eyelid skin. It is the second most common eyelid malignancy after BCC worldwide. It is an invasive malignancy arising from the squamous layer of the epithelium. It is known to cause local invasion and systemic metastasis as well.

10.3.1 Case Summary

A 75-year-old female presented with right medial canthal mass growing rapidly over last 1 year. She had undergone a lacrimal surgery which was aborted due to intraoperative identification of a firm mass. Biopsy performed revealed squamous carcinoma. On retrospect, she gave history of a small ulcerative nodule over the medial canthal skin which enlarged with bleeding over a year. Examination showed the presence of a medial canthal firm mass involving the medial lower eyelid and caruncle. The lesion was fixed to the bone and causing a mechanical ectropion and inability to open the eye completely due to fixity of mass to surrounding structures and bone. CT scan revealed the presence of eyelid and medial orbital mass invading the lacrimal sac region. Previous histopathology slides were reviewed and the diagnosis of invasive SCC was confirmed. Systemic screening including whole-body PET was normal. She underwent orbital exenteration with removal of the lacrimal sac including the nasolacrimal duct. Postoperative adjuvant radiation was given, and she is doing well at 1-year follow-up. She awaits an orbital prosthesis.

Stage	T	N	M
0	In situ	N0	M0
I	T1	N0	M0
II	T2	N0	M0
III	T3 T1 or T2	N0 or N1 N1	M0 M0
IV	T1, T2 or T3 Any T T4 Any T	N2 N3 Any N Any N	M0 M0 M0 M1

Information:

T0: No evidence of primary tumor
T1: Tumor with 2 or less cm in greatest dimension with fewer than 2 high risk features
T2: Tumor > 2 cm in greatest dimension with or without one additional high-risk features or any size with 2 or more high risk features
T3: Tumor with invasion of maxila , mandible, orbit or temporal bone
T4: Tumor with invasion of skeleton(axial or appendicular) or perineural invasion of skull bone)
N0: No regional lymph node metastasis
N1: Metastasis in single ipsilateral lymph node , 3 cm or less in greatest dimension
N2: Metastasis in single ipsilateral lymph node,> 3 cm but not > 6 cm in greatest dimension or in multiple ipsilateral lymph nodes, none > 6 cm in greatest dimension; or in bilateral or contralateral lymph nodes, none > 6 cm in greatest dimension
N2a: Metastasis in single ipsilateral lymph node, > 3cm but not > 6 cm in greatest dimension
N2b: Metastasis in multiple ipsilateral lymph nodes, none > 6 cm in greatest dimension
N2c: Metastasis in bilateral or contralateral lymph nodes, none >6cm ingreatest dimension
N3: Metastasis in lymph node, > 6cm
M0: No distant metastasis
M1: Present distant metastasis

Case 3: (**a**) Medial canthal and medial upper eyelid mass with involvement of caruncle; (**b**) CT scan showing ill-defined mass involving the orbit and lacrimal fossa; (**c**) marking for eyelid sparing exenteration; (**d**) exenterated specimen; (**e**) exenterated orbit with osteotomy for the lacrimal sac fossa and the removal of lacrimal sac; (**f**) postoperative exenterated orbit showing mild dermatitis following radiation

10.3.2 Discussion

SCC may develop de novo or certain diseases may be precursors. They are:

- Bowen's disease.
- Actinic keratosis.

Risk factors for the development of SCC are exposure to UV radiation, immunocompromised patients, human papilloma virus infection, HIV, chronic ulcers, old burns, and arsenic exposure.

Examination usually involves complete eye examination and palpation of regional lymph nodes. Usual symptoms are the presence of an ulcerative, rapidly growing lesion causing distortion of normal eyelid anatomy. Keratin may be present on some lesions. Bleeding is common from the ulcerated lesion. A full-thickness incision biopsy helps prove the diagnosis after which further treatment can be decided. SCC may vary from carcinoma in situ (CIS) to full-thickness invasive SCC which is usually determined on histopathological examination. Staging is done on the basis of American Joint Committee on staging of Cancer as shown in the table given below.

T: Tumor size
N: Nodes
M: Metastasis

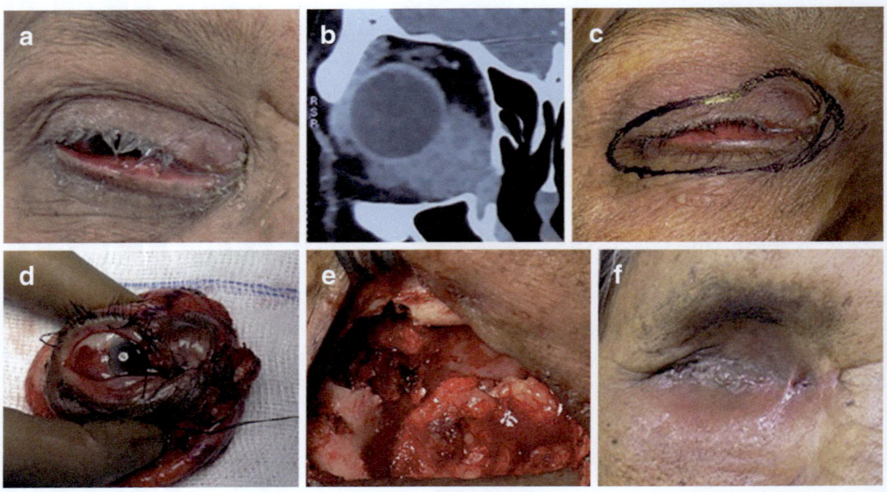

Surgical excision with wide margins is the treatment of choice. The remnant defect has to be reconstructed using skin flaps/graft. Excision using Mohs technique or frozen section prevents chances of recurrence. The presence of orbital invasion, perineural invasion, and fixity to surrounding structures warrants orbital exenteration in cases.

Poor prognostic factors include:

- Orbital spread.
- Perineural spread.
- Immunosuppression.
- Size more than 1 cm.
- Poorly differentiated tumors [1].

SCC is a highly malignant eyelid tumor which warrants prompt diagnosis and treatment. Chances of recurrence are higher than other eyelid tumors so follow-up after initial treatment is important.

Eyelid malignancies if diagnosed early have excellent prognosis with good long-term outcomes. In the Indian subcontinent, sebaceous gland carcinoma is the most common form of eyelid malignancy, and a watchful eye should be kept for masquerades of this type of eyelid tumor.

Conflict of Interest The authors have no financial interests and the photos have been displayed with proper patient consent and permission.

References

1. Lin Z, Qidwai U, Igali L, Hemmant B. A multicentre review of the histology of 1012 periocular basal cell carcinomas. Eur J Ophthalmol. 2021;31(5):2699–704.

Further Reading

Kaliki S, Bothra N, Bejjanki KM, Nayak A, Ramappa G, Mohamed A, Dave TV, Ali MJ, Naik MN. Malignant eyelid tumors in India: a study of 536 Asian Indian patients. Ocul Oncol Pathol. 2019;5(3):210–9.

Gupta R, Bhaduri A, Desai S, Das S, Menon V. Malignant tumors of the eyelid in India: a multicenter, multizone study on clinicopathologic features and outcomes. Indian J Ophthalmol. 2020;68(11):2466–70.

Cicinelli MV, Kaliki S. Ocular sebaceous gland carcinoma: an update of the literature. Int Ophthalmol. 2019;39(5):1187–97.

Sullivan TJ. Squamous cell carcinoma of eyelid, periocular, and periorbital skin. Int Ophthalmol Clin. 2009;49(4):17–24.

MIX
Papier aus verantwortungsvollen Quellen
Paper from responsible sources
FSC® C105338

If you have any concerns about our products,
you can contact us on
ProductSafety@springernature.com

In case Publisher is established outside the EU,
the EU authorized representative is:
Springer Nature Customer Service Center GmbH
Europaplatz 3, 69115 Heidelberg, Germany

Printed by Libri Plureos GmbH
in Hamburg, Germany